Rhetorical *Ethos* in Health and Medicine

This book explores rhetorical *ethos* and its ongoing role in patient credibility and in misdiagnoses stemming from gender, race and class-based biases. Drawing on the concept of *ethos* as a theoretical framework, it explores health and mental illness across different conditions and across different methodological approaches.

Extending work on *ethos* in clinical encounters and public discourse about biomedicine and presenting new research on the rhetoric of mental health, stigma and mental illness, the book explores how bias in clinical settings can mask treatable medical problems when symptoms are labelled as being "in the patient's head."

This notable contribution to the rhetoric of health and medicine will be of interest to all researchers and graduate students of rhetoric and composition studies, rhetoric of health and medicine, disability studies, medical humanities, communication, and psychology.

Cathryn Molloy is Associate Professor in James Madison University's School of Writing, Rhetoric and Technical Communication where she also serves as Director of Undergraduate Studies. Her work has appeared in *College English*, *Rhetoric Review*, *Rhetoric Society Quarterly*, *Qualitative Inquiry*, and *Technical Communication Quarterly*.

Routledge Studies in Rhetoric and Communication

For more information and a full list of titles in the series, please visit:
www.routledge.com/Routledge-Studies-in-Rhetoric-and-Communication/
book-series/RSRC

Rhetorical *Ethos* in Health and Medicine

Patient Credibility, Stigma, and Misdiagnosis

Cathryn Molloy

R Routledge
Taylor & Francis Group

LONDON AND NEW YORK

First published 2020 by Routledge

2 Park Square, Milton Park, Abingdon, Oxon OX14 4RN
605 Third Avenue, New York, NY 10017

Routledge is an imprint of the Taylor & Francis Group, an informa business

First issued in paperback 2021

Library of Congress Cataloging-in-Publication Data
A catalog record for this book has been requested

ISBN: 978-0-367-26017-0 (hbk)
ISBN: 978-1-03-217688-8 (pbk)
DOI: 10.4324/9780429291074

Typeset in Sabon
by Apex CoVantage, LLC

This book is dedicated in loving memory of
Edward K. Molloy and Sally J. Svane

Contents

Figures

Acknowledgements

I am indebted to many family members, colleagues, friends, and participants for their substantial support and help throughout the process of researching for and writing this book.

Most importantly, to all of my participants: though I do not name you specifically to protect privacy and to maintain anonymity, please know that I am grateful beyond words for your significant contributions to this work. This book would quite literally not be possible without you.

I also am deeply indebted to my graduate assistants Connor Ham and Logan Ferro for their help with research, participant recruitment, interviews, and transcriptions. Many, many thanks are also due to Nancy's Nook, Lupus Friends and Family, Celiac Disease Foundation, and Psych-Forums for their assistance with participant recruitment. I also thank the College of Physicians of Philadelphia college librarian Beth Lander for her considerable help in the archives and her exceptional patience with an inexperienced archival researcher.

For their generative and timely feedback on drafts, their guidance at various stages, and their enthusiasm for this project, I would like to express my sincerest thanks to Jen Almjeld, Rachel DiCioccio, Jeremiah Dyehouse, Ginette Ferszt, Susan Ghiaciuc, Kim Hensley-Owens, Lori Beth DeHertogh, Jenell Johnson, Molly Kessler, David LaGuardia, S. Scott Lunsford, Lisa Melonçon, Seán McCarthy, Libby Miles, Maria Novotny, Matthew Ortoleva, Alex Parrish, J. Fred Reynolds, Nedra Reynolds, Vanessa Rouillon, Bob Schwegler, Bryna Siegel-Finer, Kirk St. Amant, J. Blake Scott, Jamie White-Farnham, Jim Zimmerman, and Traci Zimmerman.

I also thank the College of Arts and Letters and the School of Writing, Rhetoric and Technical Communication (WRTC) at James Madison University and the graduate school at the University of Rhode Island (URI) for their generous support of this work in the form of grants and leave time. I thank each and every one of my supportive and collegial colleagues in WRTC and my inspiring and dedicated mentors in Writing, Rhetoric and English at URI.

An especially heartfelt thanks to my parents, sisters, and brothers for all of their love and support: Ed Molloy and Linda LaGuardia Molloy;

Irene Molloy Clancy and John Clancy; Missy Molloy and Guillaume Cailleau; Mary Molloy Cowley and Dennis Cowley; Annie Molloy Rush and Tommy Rush; John Raisch and Kathie Curtin Raisch; John Raisch and Glynis Frost Raisch; and Matthew Raisch and Jen Franklin Raisch.

Finally, I would not have been able to do this work at all without the immeasurable love and support of my family, "king accommodator" Jimmy Raisch and my beautiful boys Lucas Molloy Raisch and Mateo Molloy Raisch. Thank you so very much.

1 Introduction to Theorizing Vernacular Credibility and How Patients Mobilize *Ethos*

"You told me my pain wasn't real," wrote BuzzFeed writer Lara Parker (2017) in an open letter to a doctor who'd misdiagnosed her pain as psychogenic.[1] As she poignantly put it:

> It took me almost five years to be told that I have a disease that affects nearly 180 million people in this world. I will never get those years of my life back. . . . The ones I spent convincing myself that I belonged in a mental institution because you told me that my pain wasn't real. . . . I was suffering. And you were my only way out. But you didn't believe me."
>
> (n.p.)

Parker's story, of course, is all too common. Symptoms that evade obvious diagnosis can be erroneously dismissed as "in the patient's head" in a move that delays diagnosis and appropriate treatment, and such errors are more likely to happen to women, queer and non-binary individuals, racial/ethnic minorities, and the economically disadvantaged (Bekker & Schepman, 2009; Ladwig, Marten-Mittag, Erazo, & Gündel, 2001; Vasquez et al., 2009). Of course, these inaccurate diagnoses do quite a lot of harm to bodies and minds. Similarly, mental health struggles are often met with derision, fear, and social isolation rather than with the kinds of community accommodations and supports that might lead to better outcomes, and other marks of difference similarly exacerbate this stigma. Julian, a contributor to the "Stories" section of the Mental Health Foundation website, articulated this problem well when he described the "remarkable" impact of "discrimination and stigma" on the everyday lives of those with mental health diagnoses (Julian, 2016).

Likewise, in a piece that explored the complications with obtaining an autism diagnosis as an African American woman who doesn't "look the part," Ashley P. (2017) explained the attendant misdiagnosis of unrelated mental health disorders: "The reports would say that my life is significantly affected by the characteristics of autism. Yet I left each time with another new psychological disorder attached to my name" (n.p.).

Arguably, some of the most confounding health and medical issues exist in the milieu Parker, Julian, and Ashley succinctly illustrated above where sociopolitical realities hit up against complicated clinical presentations to create less-than-livable conditions. Indeed, "current diagnostic models in medical practice do not adequately account for patient symptoms that cannot be classified (Kornelsen, Atkins, Brownell, & Woollard, 2016, p. 367), and, as Frances (2012) pointed out, inaccurate mental health diagnoses, which are common, can be disastrous and lead "not only to inappropriate medication but also to stigma, ruined self-confidence, reduced ambition, needless worries, despair about the future, and a deeply injured sense of self" (n.p.).

Public writings like these highlight the consequences of the arbitrary fault lines between physical and mental health and between organic and psychosocial etiologies. Contested diagnoses, unexplained behaviors or symptoms, and mental disabilities that sidestep clear, consistent ameliorative interventions are adversely impacted by stigma. Relatedly, specious beliefs about a person's credibility based on demographic markers interfere with clinical judgment, and treating ailments of heads and bodies as separate and separable does not always lead to the best outcomes for patients.

These patients' stories, found online, compellingly illustrate why "the creation, circulation, and contestation of vernacular rhetoric has increased dramatically with the growth of new media" as the "opportunity for previously marginalized groups to disseminate their message has expanded" in step with "new media forms" that "offer ways to gain access, albeit constrained and controlled, to the public sphere" (Smith, 2010, p. 65). This book addresses these complex realities via vernacular engagements with rhetorical *ethos*. Rather than doing so by strictly looking in new media spaces, though, it does so by examining a variety of data that might otherwise be considered throwaway—everyday conversations, routine exchanges with doctors, and answers to a 19th century health survey. Collecting and naming everyday utterances and taking them to be serious signs of rhetorical savvy prove that, as the literature on the vernacular has made clear, there is much to be learned from looking beyond the sanctioned and/or privileged discourses for sources of new rhetorical theories.

Before going into particulars, I would like to provide some working definitions that will help frame this project. These definitions will be extended and complicated as the book moves forward, but introducing these definitions now will allow readers to start at the same place:

> *Vernacular discursive practices*: everyday, ephemeral, unofficial written and spoken communication
> *Ethos*: credibility of the speaker, both in terms of reputation and in terms of real-time performance (earned and unearned)

Kakoethos: lack of credibility or perception of poor character, both in terms of reputation and in terms of real-time performance (earned and unearned)

Stigma: negative views, often stereotypical

Implicit bias: prejudice against (or in favor of) a particular group that a person holds without conscious awareness

Anchoring bias: care providers' reluctance to consider alternative diagnoses after an initial diagnosis is made—even when new evidence suggests alternative etiologies

A major premise of this book is that rhetorical analyses of vernacular discursive practices might give way to theories that could illuminate and even alter some of the suffering associated with these dense issues. Theorizing rhetorical *ethos* (or credibility/good character) beyond earned or deserved credibility and *kakoethos* (or poor character)[2] that is neither earned nor deserved, but is based on biases, is a powerful way to frame inquiries into everyday talk and writing and their role in patient empowerment. That is, rather than focusing on official, sanctioned texts and contexts, the analyses herein focus on capturing and elevating ephemeral communications and their consequences. The book, thus, adds to expert and lay efforts to analyze complex biopsychosocial elements of human life. The chapters herein specifically demonstrate the role stigmas and biases play in clinical settings and share patients'[3] vernacular strategies, drawn from diverse empirical data, for continually building and rebuilding credibility in everyday health and medical contexts of great consequence—especially when credibility is unfairly compromised. Diverse data such as observational study, interviews, and archival material come together to present portraits of patients with a variety of mental and physical symptoms and diagnoses. Examining these strategies through which individuals with complex mental and physical health diagnoses work within and struggle against unfair, institutionalized forms of bias and attendant mistreatment, this book showcases everyday *ethos*-building and -rebuilding and their impact on patient empowerment. This chapter sets the stage for the work to come by establishing the book's goals, defining research areas under study, detailing methods while justifying their use, and briefly overviewing the theories that emerged from the studies herein.

This project enters at the intersection of a number of vibrant, interdisciplinary fields of study, including: the rhetoric of health and medicine (RHM)[4] and its branch of scholarship in mental health rhetoric research (MHRR); disability studies; the rhetoric of science (RoS); and interdisciplinary research on stigma in health and medicine. Since RHM—a relatively new field designation—might not be familiar to readers, it is worth spending some time explaining its exigencies and origins. RHM is a growing, interdisciplinary field of study marked by what Melonçon and Scott (2018b) have called "methodological mutability" or "a willingness or even obligation to pragmatically and ethically adjust aspects of methodology to the phenomena under study" (p. 1). Emphasizing critical praxis, RHM scholars bring "rhetorical inquiry (mostly in combination with other approaches) to bear on a number of health practices" (Melonçon & Scott, 2018a, p. 1). With an emphasis on rhetorical theories as capable of offering important insight into health and medical phenomena, RHM emerged out of a gap in knowledge; namely, the fact that "for many years, an often-overlooked aspect of health and medicine was the communicative dimension, that is the discourses—oral, written, visual, and technological" (Melonçon & Frost, 2015, p. 5).

In their introductory editors' note for the new *Rhetoric of Health and Medicine* journal, Melonçon and Scott[5] (2018b) identified RHM "mothers"[6] as the formidable scholars whose work made the field possible, including: McCarthy and Gerring (1994),[7] Condit (1984, 1990),[8] Wells (2010)[9] Schuster (2006),[10] Heifferon (2006),[11] Segal (2005),[12] Barton (2008),[13] Keränen (2010),[14] and Berkenkotter (2008).[15] Collectively, this robust body of work constitutes "foundational texts" of RHM by offering models for how to effectively use rhetorical lenses to meaningfully engage with health and medical phenomena in ways that add important new insight to interdisciplinary bodies of knowledge, and this book takes inspiration from and continues this work.

Recent scholarship that attests to the impressive growth of RHM include Teston (2017),[16] Arduser (2017),[17] Bloom-Pojar (2018),[18] Angeli (2018),[19] and Graham (2015).[20] These texts all "use rhetorical theory to guide inquiry and arrive at nuanced observations about the persuasive dimensions of their subjects of study" (Scott, 2017, n.p.), and this book seeks to do the same.

Beyond book-length studies, rhetoricians of health and medicine have taken up contested diagnoses, addressing what sociologist Jutel (2011) identified as a crucial issue in medical diagnostics: "a number of conditions—some common, others idiosyncratic—find their recognition thwarted by medicine. They are accepted neither by doctors nor by government or insurance companies yet are experienced by the individual as illness" (p. 77). For example, Keränen (2014) examined the contested illness Morgellons—considered "delusional parasitosis" by some and "infectious medical mystery" by others—to show that a "rhetorical approach to illness and disease calls attention to the role of language in shaping meaning and action" as "divergent stakeholders" compete for epistemological standing in discourses surrounding the disorder (p. 48). Keränen demonstrated that, much like other contested diseases, "peer-reviewed literature, internet content, and patient testimony interact to modify subtly both lay and clinical practices . . . even when the discourse communities otherwise advance radically different explanations of the nature and causes of the condition" (p. 48). Contested diagnoses are, in many ways, ideal for rhetorical analysis as rhetorical lenses can clarify these murky deliberative spaces. Studies like Keränen's connect to similar work in mental health rhetoric research (MHRR).

In MHRR, scholars have grappled with how claims based on expert knowledge undermine ephemeral, nonexpert body-mind knowledges (Berkenkotter, 2008; Emmons, 2010; Johnson, 2010; Lewiecki-Wilson, 2003; McCarthy & Gerring, 1994; Price, 2011; Prendergast, 2001; Reynolds, 2008; Reynolds & Mair, 2013; Uthappa, 2017). Reynolds (2018) compellingly sketched out the "significant body of work applying the tools and terms of rhetoric to the world of mental health" that emerged in the 1980s and continues today, if in fits and starts (p. 1). One key area of concern in MHRR literature has been rhetorical focus on the *Diagnostic and Statistical Manual of Mental Disorders* (DSM)—especially in terms of the text's authority as a source of current psychiatric research-based information on mental health diagnostics and treatment (Kelly, 2014; McCarthy & Gerring, 1994). As each iteration of the DSM proliferates diagnostic categories, as various constituents comment on the status of mental health around the globe, and as mental health-related words and phrases enter solidly and uncritically into popular lexicons, the importance of MHRR is undeniable.

Importantly, too, rhetoricians join other fields in recognizing the troubling power of the DSM. In *Saving Normal*, psychiatrist Francis (2013) remarked that the DSM:

> determines all sorts of important things that have an enormous impact on people's lives—like who is considered well and who is sick; what treatment is offered; who pays for it; who gets disability benefits; who is eligible for mental health, school, vocational, and other services; who gets to be hired for a job, can adopt a child, or pilot a plane, or qualifies for health insurance; whether a murderer is a criminal or a mental patient; what should be the damages awarded in a lawsuit; and much, much more.
>
> (p. xii)

Francis's concern is certainly well founded when it is considered next to rhetorical examinations of the DSM as a charter document for the discipline of psychiatry rather than an empirically sound diagnostic tool (McCarthy & Gerring, 1994). Indeed, the DSM's ever-expanding list of "disorders" has been a concern for rhetoricians of health and medicine for some time, and their critical scholarship makes it quite clear that the DSM is much more the result of power and persuasion than of rigorous science (Reynolds, 2008, p. 156; Reynolds, 2018). Similarly, when diagnostic categories proliferate in each successive iteration of the DSM, rhetoricians are able to point out that the use of this manual leads to pathologizing normal behaviors. As a result, nearly everyone is diagnosable with some mental health problem, and interventions meant to be helpful tend, ironically, to compound rather than alleviate suffering (Reynolds, 2008)—a phenomenon also noted, among other places, in the rhetorics of reproduction (see, for example, De Hertogh, 2015; Koerber, 2013; Owens, 2015). As well, RHM scholars have used rhetorical perspectives to lend important insight to the lived experiences of those with mental health diagnoses as well as to the multiple ontologies through which they come to be diagnosed in the first place (Johnson, 2010; Holladay, 2017; Rothfelder & Thornton, 2017; Reynolds, 2008; Uthappa, 2017). Much like this body of work, this book offers critical vantages on mental health discourses based in rhetorical theories.

In its attention to speaking across disciplinary lines and tending to competing epistemologies, this book also has origins and resonances in the rhetoric of science (RoS), which has a long history of crossover literature within RHM, particularly in works that invoke "rhetoric of science, technology, and medicine" (RSTM). Cagle's (2017) description of the often competing agendas for rhetoricians of science, technology, and medicine to either *understand* persuasion or to *achieve* persuasion is a sharp observation of the connections between RoS and RHM; she noted the importance of engaged scholarship, but also commented on the need to tend to "institutional structures that might undercut and that might support such engagement" (p. 10). Cagle's work contributed to a large corpus of meta-literature on RoS that spans decades.[21]

Much like RHM in its focus on evaluating the efficacy and justice of knowledge claims, RoS begins with the premise that "like any other powerful cultural institution, science must be watched carefully—and checked when necessary—in an effort to prevent abuses" (Zerbe, 2007, p. 2). RoS work also engages with such issues as "changed boundaries between science and its publics" and "new possibilities for public communication" (Miller, 2013); it "emphasizes that representations need to make science meaningful for diversified audiences from different academic backgrounds and cultures" (Freddi, 2013, p. 228). Moreover, much like RHM in its use of rhetorical lenses to arrive at innovative conclusions about the subject under study, RoS, much like this book, uses the "resources of the rhetorical tradition" to examine "text, tables, and visuals of the sciences" (Gross, 2008, p. 1). Likewise, this book follows RoS scholars for whom it is common to combine rhetorical inquiries with methods borrowed from the social sciences (Gross, 2008, p. 4).[22] Like Walsh's (2013) rhetorical genealogy in which she successfully uses wide-ranging archival data to suggest that scientists often make use of prophetic *ethos* in their attempts to influence public audiences who can secure funding and implement policy, this book uses *ethos* as a primary rhetorical/theoretical anchoring point. *Ethos* is a powerful lens for RoS-related inquiries since convincing audiences that "one has to speak for nature" or is able to "have nature speak through him or her" relies on a "person's ability to persuade us that he or she is a properly constituted scientist" (Segal & Richardson, 2003, p. 140).

Rather than saying that scientists set out to do harm, moreover, Walsh's analysis seeks to demystify the processes by which they arrive at scientific truths; she uses rhetoric to uncover the role that persuasion plays in the process. My analyses in this book similarly show the role *ethos* plays in rendering some rhetorical actors authorized or unauthorized to speak truths of their bodies and minds, but it does so without giving in to the temptation to devolve into ad hominem attacks on health and medical practitioners.

Noting that "in our post-critical age" some scholars have "sought to build different relationships with our colleagues in science and medicine" in the face of extreme challenges, some scholars have sought to work within the "gap" between science and the humanities (Herndl, 2017, p. 1), and this book also makes that move. An issue that comes up in RoS as well as in RHM and RSTM and related fields, of course, is the formation of disciplinary silos and attendant unintelligibility of work across disciplinary boundaries—a problem that leads to scholarly coteries or academic literature that lectures the already converted (St. Amant & Graham, 2019).

Condit (2013) argued that:

> To be an academic should not mean to find the narrowest possible community to credit or gain accreditation with. It should be to accept the mission of enhancing understanding, where understanding engages maximal possible breadth under the—necessarily and desirably vague—trajectory of improving the richness of life for human beings while protecting the natural world around us.
>
> (p. 4)

Ceccarelli (2013), too, lamented the lack of movement and influence of RoS scholarship; as she put it:

> It turns out that the central problem for rhetoricians is not that we present ourselves as overly aggressive transformers of all we survey, but that for the most part, we fail to creatively project ourselves onto horizons of possibility as forces of change at all. In articles written to each other, we find ourselves preaching to the choir, with only passing mention of our obligation to reach out to the very audiences who are empowered to make the alterations to practice that our critical findings recommend.
>
> (p. 1)

Ceccarelli, thus, calls on rhetoricians of science to take on the mission of making the work matter outside the field (p. 7). Similarly, RHM scholars must make efforts to produce scholarship that reaches those in the trenches in health and medicine, including diverse patients, caregivers, and care providers. Reaching these diverse constituents means engaging in work that is critical of systems of oppression, yet tentative and mindful of the benevolence of many healthcare workers and allowing for the possibility that some good comes from positivist epistemologies. Still, making room for critiques of positivist truth claims when they could be harmful is crucial to the success of our work. It is in this spirit that I reflect on this book's connections to the important work being done in disability studies.

While rhetoric scholars have looked closely at the language associated with health and medicine and with mental health, disability studies brings an important dimension to my study and its contributions because the field privileges the individual over the diagnosis, questions the binary between "normal" and "disabled," and focuses on the social epistemic at work in understandings of disabilities (Holladay, 2017, p. 11). The field emphasizes built environments that are disabling over and against the notion of personal defect and on accommodations and integration over isolation. Disability studies also highlights the tendency for various discourses and physical realities to advance ableism, or the idea that being temporarily able-bodied or for the time being of so-called "sound" mind is always preferable and inherently superior to that which is slated as "disabled" in a given culture. These logics at work in disability studies are tremendously empowering, generative, and important. Significant disability studies projects have advanced efforts in RHM and in writing and rhetoric more generally to ennoble stigmatized positions. Notable examples include Price (2011)[23] and Dolmage (2009, 2015, 2017).[24] This project shares disability studies' commitment to highlighting the arbitrary nature of slating certain ways of being in the world as inherently superior or even simply "normal" as such notions are highly problematic social constructions that leave out wide swaths of the human community.

Where readers will notice this project parting ways significantly with disability studies, though, is in its acceptance of biomedical frameworks— a move that is made with not only an appreciation for disability studies scholars' more radical undertakings, but also with a sense that producing scholarship that aligns epistemologically with the day-to-day work of diverse health and medical practitioners might be better poised to perform the difficult work of advocating especially for the rhetors under study who've been severely disenfranchised. There are some everyday helpful or even lifesaving health and medical practices that result from biomedical lines of argument. Those whose everyday work is with the very ill or dying need a wide variety of epistemologies. Disability studies as a discipline uncovers taken-for-granted systems of oppression that lead to uneven power dynamics and the arbitrary elevation of certain subjectivities as standard or ideal with deep and far-reaching consequences. Disability studies scholarship must often discredit biomedical frameworks to maintain the integrity of its larger aims. Their critiques bring biases and abuses to light. This book, though, allows for the possibility that some positivist notions inherent in biomedicine could be valid. The complexities that come with navigating the many ontologies at play in the subjects under study in this book require a wide spectrum of perspectives across epistemological allegiances.

This book shows how patient credibility is built on unremarkable everyday interactions that are potential sites of purposeful intervention. It takes energy from RHM, RoS and RSTM work that highlights the need to interrogate and work on the edges of the arbitrary borders between the humanities, social, and hard sciences. It advocates for productive hybrid scholarship that engages meaningfully with (rather than dismissing as irrelevant) basic epistemological assumptions of other disciplines.[25]

It, thus, relies quite heavily on interdisciplinary mental health research on stigma and on misdiagnosis due to demographics, and those areas of emphasis warrant an entire chapter to unpack, which make them the subject of Chapter 2. RHM is inherently interdisciplinary, and this project is no exception. Its chapters' major moves rely on biomedicine and studies of biomedical discourses; still, they follow disability studies with attention to tacit and overt forms of everyday unfairness that go largely unrecognized by the general public. As the fields of study to which this book relates make clear, "a rhetorical approach not only intersects with, but also provides potential contributions to, qualitative inquiry" (Endres, Hess, Senda-Cook, & Middleton, 2016, p. 512), and methods and methodologies selected follow that logic. Before delving into those methods and methodologies, I'll first overview important theories.

Overview of Important Theories

This book argues for the value of *ethos* as a generative lens through which to compose important new theories in a variety of health and medical contexts and beyond. These theories are meant to pay homage to disenfranchised persons' impressive, everyday rhetorical performances and to suggest that others might adapt similar discursive behaviors on their own behalf. Importantly, rhetorical *ethos* offers a lens through which scholars might strategically examine who is believed, in what contexts, and why. Such information is crucial as it allows for the possibility of building theories through which those who aren't believed and, thus, suffer myriad social, emotional, and physical consequences, might build, recover and bolster their credibility in the various health and medical (or medicalized) contexts they face. As well, elevating disenfranchised rhetors' everyday rhetorical strategies does important epistemological work as it advances the status of their rhetorical significance. *Ethos* is decidedly not a static entity; it is constantly in the state of being made and remade. Within new materialist frameworks, such as Graham's (2015) "rhetorical-ontological inquiry" in its "aim to place the material and the ontological at the center of inquiry" (p. 7), it becomes possible to recognize the power of human and nonhuman forces to shape and reshape everyday realities. Similarly, I use *ethos* in a dynamic sense and offer insight into different ways patients mobilize *ethos* in everyday contexts. I consider, for example, bodily performances alongside speech acts to describe appeals to *ethos*, and I analyze, to the extent possible given the data, the efficacy of those appeals.

Ethos, of course, refers most commonly to "credibility of the speaker," and Amossy (2001) offered a succinct and clear discussion of the two competing theories of *ethos* that dominate much of recorded history: *ethos* as the reputation of the speaker that precedes the oratorical scene or *ethos* as discursively constructed in the context of a rhetorical performance via, for instance, a display of rhetorical competence (Hyde, 2014, p. 1). Danisch (2017) reminded readers that *ethos* in Aristotelian iterations, referred not to immutable characteristics of the speaker as in Quintilian's "good man speaking well" or in the writings of Isocrates where reputation would also be a factor, but to a *techne*: a "set of rules for meeting the constraints of the agency of the audience-as-judge in order to actualize the potential power of rhetoric in the communal, shared interactions of writer and audience" (p. 69). Brinton (1986) echoed Perelman and Olbrechts-Tyteca (1971) in delineating the ways that *ethos* in rhetoric is analogous to ad hominem in dialectic. Indeed, *ethos*, argued Segal and Richardson (2003), "refers both to the individual's character and to the social mores of her society"; it is concerned with "whether any individual has a good or bad character" as it is assessed "relative to socially available standards" (p. 141).

Though studies that take up *ethos* do not always make mention of it, any methodology for putting *ethos* to use as a compelling contemporary analytic framework must contend meaningfully with the dichotomous nature of *ēthotic* history, and most do so implicitly by insinuating that *ethos* is both the reputation that the speaker brings to the oratorical scene *and* the discursive construction of credibility in the persuasive act itself. Lesser known is *ethos* in pre-Aristotelian terms: as dwelling place. Hyde (2014) showed that the temporal dimension of *ethos* suggested by its origins in "dwelling place" allows for the possibility of reconciling the two positions on *ethos*, as

> the genuine enhancement of public opinion requires, among other things, that the orator "modify" the lived and attuned space of others by "making present" to them what the orator has reason to believe is true, just, and virtuous. In so doing, the orator not only places his own character on the line and in the text but also clears a place in time and space for people to acknowledge and "know-together" (conscientia) what is arguably the truth of some matter of importance.
>
> (p. 2)

I would argue that even scholars in mental health rhetoric and related research who are not invoking *ethos* as dwelling place do so obliquely in the ways they frame their contributions. Uthappa (2017), for example, noted that "the cultural stigmatization of mental disability guarantees that the challenge to a speaker's credibility begins the minute she reveals her condition," but also argued that those with diagnoses of mental illnesses might improve damaged *ethos* via "deep disclosure" of such diagnoses in face-to-face oral performances in which speakers gain proximity to their audiences via the vulnerability inherent in such utterances (p. 165). Similarly, Rothfelder and Thornton (2017) identified the temporal engagements through which a writer with obsessive-compulsive disorder (OCD) "plays with proximity" in a move to disorient readers (p. 378). Other studies in rhetoric also engage with *ethos* as dwelling place in compelling ways without necessarily acknowledging (or, perhaps, without awareness of) the origins of the *"ethos* as dwelling place" vantage point, such as Bordelon's (2016) focus on embodiment, location, and accretion in her analysis of the Delsarte system of acting, which she used to showcase *ethos* as expressed "through and by means of the body" (p. 105). These projects showcase the affordances of using *ethos* as a framing mechanism for powerful inquiries, and this book similarly highlights the dynamic nature of *ethos* as an embodied appeal that is constantly in flux.

Focusing on *ethos* in health and medicine, of course, isn't new, and this book takes inspiration from other RHM work on *ethos*. Anderson's (1989) early text *Richard* Selzer *and the Rhetoric of Surgery* examined how Selzer's writings created an *ethos* and professional identity. As Segal (2005) explained, Anderson's work put forward the idea of "traditional medical rhetoric as 'vertical'; it is a rhetoric of persuasion that descends from the physician as actor to the patient as acted upon, a rhetoric that, he says, may deprive patients of their voices in 'the healing dialogue'" (Segal, 2005, p. 85). Segal further explored *ethos* in health and medicine by examining Merton's concept "sociological ambivalence" as it is "built into the structure of social statuses and roles—especially professional ones" (p. 143).

Asserting the extensive power of this professional credibility, Segal commented: "The appeal for *ethos* may, in fact, carry a medical journal article when the appeal from scientific logos fails" (Segal, 2005, p. 88). Keränen (2010) similarly put forward a three-part framework for analyzing "contested characterizations" in biomedical controversies; that framework involves considerations of *ethos*, persona, and voice (p. 21). She explained *ethos* as "persuasion through the character of the speaker" and, as such, *ethos* can often propel scientific knowledge" since when a scientist is "well known and widely respected," she can "advance her knowledge claims with more ease than one who is unknown or mistrusted—regardless of the actual content of the claims each makes" (Keränen, 2010, p. 25). Aligned well with vernacular rhetorics and with

RoS, sociologist Gieryn's (1999) work on "credibility contests" also posited that science gains credibility once it begins to circulate in everyday discursive spaces rather than simply when it is in the laboratory.

Popham (2014) likewise pointed out a "métis-like fluidity" in "*ethos* created by the therapists and social workers in the electronic charts," which was marked by "fluid oscillation" (p. 336). This *ethos*, argued Popham, is, like scientific *ethos* "objective, disinterestedly neutral, and attempts to use scientific reasoning," but it is also "unscientific in that it is author-centered and savvy in its choice of topics" as it "attempts to be the crafty and moral expert" (p. 336). Popham believed that the care providers' practices of vacillating between scientific and unscientific appeals to *ethos* are done in response to insecurities about their professional status.

That is, since social workers are not always the most valued of frontline mental healthcare providers, Popham (2014) found that the writers of juvenile mental health electronic records oscillated between a traditionally scientific/objective *ethos* and the moralizing "blame shifter" of the social worker (p. 334) Framing the charts as "rhetorical documents" that manage to "strengthen the *ethos* of the therapists/social workers as professionals" (Popham, 2014, p. 342), Popham's study makes an important contribution to studies of *ethos* in health and medicine in its use of *métis*, or cunning, to explicate the appeals to *ethos* used. Like Popham, Chapter 4 relies on *métis* to strengthen and clarify analysis of *ethos*. Taking energy and inspiration from these studies of *ethos*, this book emphasizes patient rather than provider credibility. It also relies particularly on the theories of everyday or vernacular *ethos*. In fact, a vernacular approach to *ethos* is a crucial part of this book's methodology.

Methods and Methodologies

In this book, the complex entanglements in which vernacular rhetorics live and move are foregrounded by elevating ephemeral exchanges to the level of texts worth serious study. The chapters in this book make use of a methodology that, "in the pursuit of understanding and interpreting everyday and mundane rhetorics," relies on "qualitative research" and, thus, "incorporates tenets of interviewing, participant observation, and fieldwork into rhetorical criticism" (Endres et al., 2016, p. 515). The focus on everyday tactics to build credibility honors the flux with which health and medical realities unfold, and this focus is meant to mitigate a "side effect of the use of written illness narratives," which is the "sense of the narrative as singular and frozen in time" (Goldstein, 2015, p. 133).

The vantage this book takes in relation to patient credibility and *ethos*, moreover, is best captured in the spirit of the "rhetorics of the vernacular" and "rhetorics of the everyday"[26] movements, which create "ear to the ground optics" (Goldstein, 2015, p. 138). In the same way, the data I examine in Chapters 3, 4, and 5 elevate everyday rhetors' vernacular discursive practices, treating their ephemeral utterances and verbal or written recollections as important artifacts worthy of serious rhetorical study. A deeper look at vernacular rhetoric scholarship will make this connection and the value of such work clearer.

Examining the French philosophic 1980s contingent responsible for the influx of interest in the everyday, Vaughan-Williams and Stevens (2016) commented that interdisciplinary scholars have been "influenced by the diverse works of thinkers such as Henri Lefebvre, Michel de Certeau and Karl Barthes" and that "this heterogeneous body of work finds common ground in giving greater importance to the quotidian: to the 'spaces, rhythms, objects, and practices' around us" (p. 44). Studies of the vernacular, thus, consider the often invisible, tacit, difficult-to-track role disenfranchised entities of various kinds play in shaping sociopolitical realities.[27]

A key feature of vernacular rhetorical work and vernacular scholarship in general, then, is that it gets at what is missed when inquiries focus on official, sanctioned, permanent or semipermanent discourses that draw authority from traditional and/or institutional power structures. In some ways, conceptually, the vernacular is definable by its opposites; it is that which is not "specialized, official, institutional, learned, or elite" (Ingraham, 2013, p. 2). The vernacular gestures to the vast network of regularly overlooked human and nonhuman rhetors worth exploring. Examining the vernacular implicitly argues that it "must not be cast aside as trivial" and that it should, instead, "be embraced as the rhetorical embodiment of a larger social structure within which it operates" since "one-way transmission of 'official rhetoric'" does not offer the same analytic affordances (McClellan, 2011, p. 196).[28]

Although the connection is most often implicit, the scholarship on vernacular and everyday rhetorics relates quite heavily to *doxa*, or popular opinion. Comparing *doxa* to the "ocean's undertow," Amossy (2002) explained that, much like vernacular rhetoric, *doxa* is "a forceful current, doing powerful inventional work beneath the surface of discourse" (p. 428). In a formulation that gestures toward *doxa*, sociologists Adorjan, Christensen, Kelly, and Pawluch (2012) argued that a "vernacular resource" might lead to "refocusing attention on generic processes of reality construction" (p. 470). Troup's (2009) argument that vernacular discourse is a "major factor in the formation of public opinion—particularly a form of public opinion through which people test ideas and make public judgments" also described vernacular rhetoric in ways that resemble *doxa* (p. 449).

The presence and influence of *doxa*, then, is not always immediately apparent to social actors, but it does tremendous epistemological and ideological work at the backdrop of many deliberative scenes. The analyses in this book follow these logics of *doxa* since I assume, for example, that rhetors' everyday utterances do important rhetorical work in the context of, and in opposition to, popular opinions.

Importantly, this book uses "vernacular" and "everyday" interchangeably and uses both terms in line with explorations of *doxa* since vernacular rhetorics create and are often manifestations of often overlooked, yet powerful *doxa*. As Gibbons (2014) demonstrated in her astute read of the Dr. Spock baby care books as allowing Freudian thought to infiltrate popular opinion on human development in ways that led those who've never read Freud to hold beliefs that align with his theories, *doxa* can have origins in sanctioned discourses, yet those starting points are largely unacknowledged. In the same way, the analyses of everyday rhetorical acts examined in this book operate from the logics of *doxa*—that popular opinions are heavily influenced by and profoundly manipulate everyday exchanges. Thus, in Chapter 3, for example, popular opinions on women's propensities to have symptoms "in their heads" lead to myriad problems for the medically ill, and these rhetors' everyday acts of self-advocacy via appeals to *ethos* reframe that misconception.

Like other scholars of the vernacular, too, I rely on "ongoing exchanges of ordinary people rather than leaders for an understanding of issues" such that these "ordinary exchanges" might "define issues and construct rhetorically salient meanings" (Hauser, 2011, p. 169). I, thus, hope this book might provide "deep insight" into what is missed when rhetorical studies focus "exclusively on the formal rhetoric of leaders" (Hauser & McClellen, 2009, p. 26). Using the rhetorical choices of "historically marginalized communities" (Phillips, 2012, p. 263), such as those with chronic mental health diagnoses and contested conditions, this book provides "more raw and revealing" findings than "official or formal rhetorical counterparts considered alone" (Hauser, 2011, p. 169).

In these ways, the book attempts "to uncouple vernacular knowledge from the assumption that it is trickle-down science" (Fissell, 2006, p. 6) by arguing that the everyday rhetorical moves that rhetors without a lot of power make nonetheless have an impact on the world that is worth theorizing.

It is quite possible to study the vernacular from a one-dimensional, alphabetic text perspective. However, giving consideration to the everyday means paying attention to multimodality.[29] Considering everyday rhetorics rather than focusing on traditional rhetorical texts calls attention to the fact that "arguments—and even language—may not be the fundamental grounds of persuasion" (Muckelbauer, 2016, p. 37). Similar to rhetorical ethnography, vernacular rhetorical inquiries are implicitly multimodal or even new materialist/object-oriented in their ontologies. There is "a rich culture of vernacular media expression," and "critical discourse rooted in the cultural margins" often circulate "through these production practices" (Aguayo, 2016, n.p.).

Focusing on vernacular or everyday rhetorics, thus, works well with a consideration of "the difficulty in teasing apart . . . things, technologies, objects, animals, etc." from humans; such studies make it clear that "things are rhetorical" (Barnett & Boyle, 2016, p. 1). While this book does not go deeply into new materialist ontologies, it does complicate the notion of the vernacular as purely linguistic by examining embodied practices as appeals to *ethos*. Attention to multimodal aspects of vernacular inquiry add to other discourses on its scope and importance.

Arguing that vernacular discourse should be criticized with the same rigor of official texts, Ono and Sloop (1995) commented that it is not enough to locate and catalogue vernacular texts. Instead, scholars must bring "critical suspicion, the kind of suspicion that rhetoricians have always given mainstream discourse" to vernacular objects such that the development of new frameworks is possible (p. 21). They, thus, highlighted the need to avoid fetishizing the vernacular in ways that only offset and undermine its contributions.

The chapters in this book, likewise, use the vernacular focus alongside rhetorical terms to illuminate what might otherwise be buried or missed and to honor what Hauser and McClellen (2009) described as the value of accounting for the theoretical riches of "counterpublic and subaltern spheres" (p. 29). Much like Spivak's (1988) work on the subaltern, though, there is a tentativeness to the findings as the vernacular discursive practices I gain access to are necessarily tainted by my presence—a limitation I unpack more in Chapter 6.

Of course, methodologies of the vernacular and of the everyday cross over into rhetorical ethnographic work (explicated more in Chapter 5) and feminist research methodologies (examined further in Chapter 4) in their commitments to undervalued or underrepresented data and analyses. The connection between the vernacular and ethnography is well documented as "critical-rhetorical ethnography offers rhetorical scholars a method for seeking out and working within local and vernacular discourses" (Hess, 2011, p. 148).

This book also pays homage to feminist rhetorical research methodologies—particularly in its approaches to ethics. Feminist rhetoricians have shown sustained concern for ethics in research methods, and feminist ideologies elucidate best practices (Kirsch, 2005). Interdisciplinary qualitative health researchers have also contributed to robust literature on the topic of vulnerable research participants and ethics (Dhai, 2017; Harris, 2015; Porr, Drummond, & Olson, 2012; Van Delden & Van der Graaf, 2016) From this body of work, I've adapted important ways to weigh risk versus benefit in qualitative research (Opsal et al., 2016).

In line with feminist research methodologies, too, I admit that it is impossible for me to fully distance my "physical, emotional, professional and embodied selves" from this work, so I use these selves "as a research tool to attend to and analyze emotion, interpret data and build rapport and a sense of common understanding with the participant during fieldwork" such that "acts of reciprocity and caring, engaging active listening and showing emotion and empathy or being supportive" common in feminist research methods are heavy presences in this book (Carroll, 2013, p. 548). The methodological approaches this book takes, then, consider "affect seriously," since "the personal-ethico-political becomings of analysis cannot be easily separated out into a mechanical process of coding," and I openly acknowledge that "the knowledge produced" in this book is profoundly "affectively situated" (Ringrose & Renold, 2014). Readers will, thus, encounter affect in tone and content.

More specifically, in an attempt to further efforts in RHM, disability studies, and RoS to simultaneously move beyond disciplinary silos and toward innovative solutions to complex health and medical problems, this book uses a variety of research methods that are anchored in a focal through line in vernacular and everyday rhetorics.[30] To that end, I use methods—interviews, observations, archival materials[31]—with features of grounded theory where the "grounding" is in everyday appeals to rhetorical *ethos*. While Chapters 3, 4, and 5 discuss grounded theory to showcase how it is used with specific data, it is worth noting here that "the name 'grounded theory' mirrors its fundamental premise that researchers can and should develop theory from rigorous analyses of empirical data," and that the procedures that grounded theory practitioners follow involve "coding data; developing, checking, and integrating theoretical categories; and writing analytic narratives throughout inquiry" (Charmaz & Belgrave, 2015, p. 1). Theories developed via "grounded" methods are often middle-range theories, or what sociologist Merton (1968) described as "between the minor hypotheses of day to day research and unified theory" (p. 39). Importantly, "middle range level is below the more philosophical or grand theories and above empirical generalizations framed as hypotheses" (Liehr & Smith, 2017, p. 51). As such, middle theories are tentative and malleable—a strength I exploit by calling on other researchers to adapt, morph, and enhance the theories developed here for their own projects. That is, using a variety of methods to unpack issues with misdiagnosis and stigma in health, medicine, and mental health under the single methodology of everyday or vernacular *ethos* with grounded theory as a guiding principle allows me to use diverse vernacular participant data to develop new theories of *ethos* that might inform future study.

Chapter Summaries

The chapters in this book specifically rely on rhetorical *ethos* to interrogate unexplained symptoms; contested and delayed diagnoses; and psychosocial health and medical phenomena. Through examining the firsthand experiences of those who'd been misdiagnosed with symptoms "in their heads" prior to accurate physical disease diagnoses, the experiences of those whose phantom limb pain had been largely misunderstood as psychogenic, and the experiences of those with serious mental health diagnoses navigating an outpatient care setting, the chapters explore the landscape of contested medical diagnoses, somatic symptom disorder, and mental health diagnoses as microcosms of what *ethos* can offer inquiries into the communicative dimensions of health and medicine.

Chapter 2 continues the argument begun in this chapter, that rhetorical *ethos* is a highly generative framework for investigating the roles stigmas and abuses play in patterns of persuasion as they relate to social reproduction. The majority of the chapter explores existing literature and related media texts that exemplify the kinds of stigmas and biases that mark health and medical care. The chapter focuses on such issues as implicit bias and anchoring bias. Implicit bias, again, is a form of bias based on race, class, and/or gender that informs care decisions, but is often at odds with care providers' stated ideologies. Anchoring bias names the phenomenon by which physicians become fixated on an initial diagnosis such that they are less likely to notice or acknowledge clinical information that contradicts that decision.

Chapter 3 relies on 68 interviews with a diverse group of men and women from around the world[32] who convey remarkable stories of contested psychiatric diagnoses and years-long bouts of suffering before obtaining accurate diagnoses of physical disease. Journalist Dusenbery's (2018) new monograph *Doing Harm: The Truth About How Bad Medicine and Lazy Science Leave Women Dismissed, Misdiagnosed, and Sick* contributed to a burgeoning body of narrative work on patient mistreatment in mainstream health and medical contexts, and Chapter 3 extends and challenges this area of inquiry by avoiding critiquing healthcare providers and focusing, instead, on patient's empowering rhetorical moves for undermining biases in clinical settings. That is, this chapter uses data from diverse participants to suggest that everyday discursive behaviors might bolster *ethos* and make accurate diagnoses more likely. Interview data are used to develop theories on how these linguistic choices might be theorized and clarified. Rhetoric scholars—in the business of examining how expert knowledges are touted as immutable truths in moves to shut down deliberation and to undermine everyday, nonexpert epistemologies—are uniquely positioned to contribute to conversations on misdiagnoses of psychogenic symptoms. Chapter 3, thus, focuses on how patients use rhetorical tactics to overcome care providers' claims that symptoms are psychogenic, but it also suggests that patients' everyday talk is fertile ground for new rhetorically informed theories.

Chapter 4, then, examines American Civil War amputees' tacit strategies for reasserting their full personhood following the stigmatizing experiences of wartime limb loss through an analysis of surveys they completed decades after amputation. I examined these surveys in 19th century physician S. Weir Mitchell's papers, which are housed in the Philadelphia College of Physicians archives. These men's experiences with stigma stem not only from their status of less-than-fully-human in the eyes of their

19th century contemporaries, but also from their claims to maintaining feeling in their missing limbs or "phantom limb pain" (PLP)—a condition once very much believed to be a psychological manifestation and more recently found to have physical, neurological causes. Like American Civil War amputees, contemporary veterans worldwide with marks of difference, such as physical or mental disability, are unfairly stigmatized and, thus, considered unreliable, and Chapter 4 ends with a meditation on how these archival materials suggest the consequences of ignoring disenfranchised veterans' self-knowledges.

Of course, using PLP to draw attention to the enigmatic nature of pain in its various states of being tacitly addresses somatic symptoms and, thus, a direct line is drawn from the investigations conducted in Chapter 3 to the objects of inquiry in Chapter 4. If pain can be experienced in a body part that no longer remains attached to the body, the idea that the sensation could have organic etiologies would seem impossible to support. Thus, space opens to consider pain a subjective experience of suffering that is at least partially "in your head." That is the conundrum I believe these veterans were in when they tried to explain their experiences of PLP. Chapter 4 shares how these men were ahead of their time. In fact, their descriptions of PLP as having physical and psychological causes—moves to legitimate their suffering—align quite well with current clinical knowledge.

Chapter 5[33] presents two concepts I developed through ethnographic research at an outpatient facility for those with chronic mental health diagnoses: "recuperative *ethos*" and "agile epistemologies." Recuperative *ethos* refers to the "day-to-day discursive practices through which a person might regain credibility and, as a consequence, rebuild the personal, social, and professional standing that is often compromised in acute phases of mental illnesses" (Molloy, 2015, p. 140). Agile epistemologies are "intriguing, inventive vernacular rhetorical performances that evoke an embodied experience of nimbleness . . . these quick-witted utterances performed meaning-making through language and gestures" (Molloy, 2015, p. 146). Recuperative *ethos* and agile epistemologies use everyday talk as a potent source of new rhetorical theories. This chapter ends with a call for researchers to adapt these terms for their own projects, as Thorvilson and Copeland (2018) successfully did in their study of parents' strategies for establishing their credibility following the diagnosis of Trisomy 18 in their infants.

The final chapter, "Toward a Methodology for Studying Everyday *Ethos* in Clinical Settings," offers up a methodology for future study of credibility in a variety of health and medical contexts where this ancient rhetorical concept might illuminate complex problems that plague contemporary life around the globe. Rather than suggesting that this work be done via strict adherence to existing theories, the chapter advocates an openness to using vernacular or everyday utterances to build new theories with the capacity to continue to adapt to a stream of new contexts and data sources as they emerge.

In sum, this book is an interdisciplinary project in RHM that takes up credibility or rhetorical *ethos* as a particularly relevant framing mechanism for interrogating the role stigmas and abuses play in patterns of persuasion as they relate to social reproduction in health and medicine. This book showcases the value of rhetorically focused humanities projects for unpacking especially thorny health and medical realities. This project, thus, adds to scholarship that takes up a "rhetorical approach to illness and disease" as it "call[s] attention to the role of language in shaping meaning and action" (Keränen, 2014, p. 48). Of course, many more studies are needed on the role rhetorical *ethos* plays in complex, subjective interchanges between care providers and patients (and those deemed "patients" and their everyday interlocuters),[34] and this book is limited in scope to stigmas that accompany psychiatric diagnoses and misdiagnoses of physical conditions as psychological problems. It is my hope that this book will serve as a methodological model for future projects that will take up the universal issue of credibility in clinical exchanges and beyond from many more vantage points.

As Scott, Segal, and Keränen (2013) have suggested, "If our work is to fulfill its aims, it must reach and influence its multiple audiences, which include the range of stakeholders and publics tied to the practices we examine" (p. 3). Much like the work in MHRR suggests, RHM is poised to work across disciplines on projects that take more explicitly activist roles. RHM work can be used to advocate for more prudence and transparency in diagnostic practices; it can have a hand in ending stigma associated with certain diagnoses (via increasing patient agency and *ethos*). RHM provides the tools to work within etiological uncertainties and the attendant tensions between illnesses as lived experiences of distress and diseases as organically verifiable complaints. This book takes up vernacular epistemologies via diverse methods to carve out space for and to argue in favor of an expansive methodology for studying *ethos* in contemporary health and medical contexts with a specific emphasis on the usefulness of *ethos* as a terministic screen[35] for unpacking contested health and medical realties not only at the backdrop of real-time discursive behaviors, but also in the temporally rich kairotics moments in which speakers argue—both tacitly and directly—for their credibility.

Notes

1. Psychogenic symptoms are physical sensations that are believed to be the result of psychiatric and/or emotional distress.
2. See Johnson (2010) for a discussion of *kakoEthos*, or "bad character."
3. I use "patient" here not to privilege the medical gaze, but to call attention to the fact that the discourses examined in the chapters in this book are contextually

linked by the fact that participants are discussing or performing in care settings and/or are reflecting on such performances.

4. In RHM, scholars are purposefully carving out space for work that explicitly engages in "rhetorical theorizing and analysis" (Melonçon & Scott, 2018, p. 4). While this scholarly area "has a longer history under different names" such as, but not limited to, "health communications" (Melonçon & Frost, 2015, p. 8), "medical rhetoric," "rhetoric of medicine," or "biomedical rhetoric" (Scott, Segal, & Keränen, 2013, p. 1), the move to call the field by a specific name addressed the fact that this kind of scholarship had been difficult to identify as a discrete corpus due to diverse nomenclature. The lack of cohesion led Scott, Segal, and Keränen (2013) to implore scholars to use the common phrase "rhetoric of health and medicine" to describe the work they are doing, and, thus, to streamline scholars' efforts to find and engage with related work in their own original health and medical rhetorics projects.

5. The field of RHM owes a debt of gratitude to Melonçon and Scott, whose tireless work to create a "dwelling place" for the field in the new journal among other places will inevitably lead to more cohesion and more participation.

6. Likewise, Melonçon and Scott's writings make it clear that RHM is an implicitly feminist activist scholarly space as there are no "seminal" texts, but foundational texts that emerge from the efforts of women scholars.

7. Field-based research on a DSM revision.

8. Women's healthcare rights and embodiment.

9. Study of rhetoric and *Our Bodies, Ourselves*.

10. Work on rhetoric and/of midwifery.

11. Work on rhetoric and/of smallpox.

12. Landmark volume *Health and the Rhetoric of Medicine*.

13. Work in medical ethics.

14. Study of trust in medical discourse.

15. Work on case histories in psychiatry.

16. Study of medical uncertainty in cancer care wherein she highlights the human and nonhuman flux that constitute health and medical evidence.

17. Study of diabetes as a chronic condition that, thus, necessitates a new, rhetorically informed concept of agency that is patient-centered.

18. Ethnographic study of a summer health program in Dominican Republic that charts the relationship between dialectal variation and power in health exchanges.

19. Study of the on-the-spot rhetorical decision-making of emergency medical services professionals.

20. Rhetorical-ontological inquiry into pain medicine that both defines and uses a hybrid methodological approach to studying health and medical phenomena by drawing on a variety of data sources to unpack the various "ontologies" of pain.

21. See, for example, Ceccarelli (2001), Gross (1996), Fahnestock (2005), Herndl & Cutlip (2013), Johnson (2014), White (2014).

22. Other scholars argued for RoS as a crucial area of study by delineating its aims. Remarking on a review study of RoS scholarship, Condit (2013) mentioned three major categories in RoS beyond theory-building: "to challenge specific representations associated with science," to explore "the relative influence of science on public policies," and to provide "Isocratean" studies that offer to improve scientific rhetorics (p. 2).

23. Explicitly brings disability studies frameworks to bear on issues of mental disability in the academy to highlight the ways that existing institutional structures and dominant dispositions unfairly marginalize those labelled mentally disabled.

24. Critiques ableism in the academy and calls on readers to recognize the central place of disability in higher education. Foregrounds the need to incorporate aspects of universal design into curricular decision-making for college students. Argues that imagining and using feedback from the most diverse group of students in terms of abilities inevitably improves instruction for everyone.

25. This book also relates to research on clinical conversations in health communication, and that area of emphasis is discussed at length in Chapter 3.

26. Importantly, I use "everyday" and "vernacular" interchangeably.

27. These studies have origins in rhetorical scholarship that marks and tracks the historic emergence of interest in and elevation of local, non-Latin languages, such as Mann's (2012) book-length archival study of English Renaissance humanism and rhetoricians' purposeful elevation of the English language—just one notable example of many projects that explore the rise of elevated vernaculars in Europe, often in the service of nationalism (p. 153). As the literature on the rhetorical dimensions of the vernacular has moved forward, it has focused more on "the process by which the lowest and the highest memorable voicings and revoicings are drawn upon" (Abrahams, 2005, p. 12) since vernacular rhetoric "is a dialectical term denoting the local rhetorics of everyday, common folk: how they speak, how they interact, what discourse informs their daily routines in the communities and places they live and work, and how these communities and places likewise inform their discourse" (Ingraham, 2013, p. 2).

28. For example, in an effort to unpack "how citizens conceptualize and experience 'threat' and '(in)security'" beyond large-scale studies of public opinion (p. 41), Vaughan-Williams and Stevens (2016) conducted focus group research across six British cities to "argue that vernacular constructions, experiences and stories of (in)security have the potential to disrupt 'official' accounts and repoliticize the technocratic foundations of national security policies" (p. 42). That is, examining everyday citizens' interpretations of their security needs in real time offered the researchers ways to productively interrogate top-down ways of understanding citizens' beliefs and needs. Like other studies of the vernacular, "authority" for meaning-making in Vaughan-Williams and Stevens' work "need not be granted based on participation solely in communities driven by expertise or locality" (Bennett, 2014, p. 216).

29. Indeed, vernacular discourses are composed of components of community, such as "the music, art, criticism, dance, and architecture of local communities," and are "unique to specific communities" (Ono & Sloop, 1995, p. 20).

30. Interestingly, Vaughan-Williams and Stevens noted a distinction between those who favor "vernacular" as "working within" the "high/low" and "elite/everyday" politics binaries and those who prefer "everyday" working in opposition to that binary (p. 44). That trend is not something I noted in the literature where most use the terms interchangeably, so I do the same.

31. Archival research methodologies will be explored in Chapter 4.

32. Chapter 2 will offer a precise breakdown of participant demographics and will make it clear that most participants are from the US.

33. This chapter is derived, in part, from an article published in *Rhetoric Society Quarterly* on April 3, 2015, available online: www.tandfonline.com/doi/abs/10.1080/02773945.2015.1010125.

34. Chapter 3 engages related health communications literature.

35. Kenneth Burke (1966) describes "terministic screens" as a concept to account for the fact that the "nature of our terms affect the nature of our observations" (p. 46). By calling rhetorical *Ethos* a terministic screen suitable for the examination of confounding health and medical realities, I'm signaling its usefulness for marking certain critical vantage points on these phenomena.

References

Abrahams, R. D. (2005). *Everyday life: A poetics of vernacular practices*. Philadelphia, PA: University of Pennsylvania Press.

Adorjan, M., Christensen, T., Kelly, B., & Pawluch, D. (2012). Stockholm syndrome as vernacular resource. *The Sociological Quarterly*, *53*(3), 454–474. doi:10.1111/j.1533-8525.2012.01241.x.

Aguayo, A. (2016). The bodies that push the buttons matter: Vernacular digital rhetoric as a form of communicative agency. *Enculturation*. Retrieved from http://enculturation.net/the-bodies-that-push-the-buttons-matter

Amossy, R. (2001). *Ethos* at the crossroads of disciplines: Rhetoric, pragmatics, sociology. *Poetics Today*, *22*(1), 1–23. doi:10.1215/03335372-22-1-1.

Amossy, R. (2002). Introduction to the study of doxa. *Poetics Today*, *23*(3), 369–394. doi:10.1215/03335372-23-3-369.

Anderson, C. M. (1989). *Richard Selzer and the rhetoric of surgery*. Carbondale, IL: Southern Illinois University Press.

Angeli, E. L. (2018). *Rhetorical work in emergency medical services: Communicating in the unpredictable workplace*. New York: Routledge.

Ashley, P. (2017). Did my autism fly under the radar because of my race? Retrieved from https://themighty.com/2017/11/minority-patients-and-undiagnosed-autism/

Barnett, S., & Boyle, C. (2016). *Rhetoric, through everyday things*. Tuscaloosa: University of Alabama Press.

Barton, E. (2008). Further contributions from the ethical turn in composition/rhetoric: Analyzing ethics in interaction. *College Composition and Communication*, *59*(4), 596–632.

Bekker, M. H. J., & Schepman, R. (2009). Somatization and psychological awareness of ethnic minority clients in Western-European mental health care: A pilot study. *European Journal of Psychiatry*, *23*(3), 135–139. doi: 10.4321/S0213-61632009000300001.

Bennett, J. (2014). *Born this way: Queer vernacular and the politics of origins*. Routledge. doi:10.1080/14791420.2014.924153.

Berkenkotter, C. (2008). *Patient tales: Case histories and the uses of narrative in psychiatry*. Columbia: University of South Carolina Press.

Bloom-Pojar, R. (2018). *Translanguaging outside the academy: Negotiating rhetoric and healthcare in the Spanish Caribbean*. Urbana, IL: National Council of Teachers of English.

Bordelon, S. (2016). Embodied *ethos* and rhetorical accretion: Genevieve Stebbins and the Delsarte system of expression. *Rhetoric Society Quarterly*, *46*(2), 105. doi:10.1080/02773945.2016.1141347.

Brinton, A. (1986). Ēthotic argument. *History of Philosophy Quarterly*, *3*(3), 245–258.

Burke, K. (1966). *Language as symbolic action: Essays on life, literature, and method*. Los Angeles: University of California Press.

Cagle, L. (2017). Becoming "forces of change": Making a case for engaged rhetoric of science, technology, engineering, and medicine. *Poroi*, *12*(2), n.p. doi:10.13008/2151-2957.1260.

Carroll, K. (2013). Infertile? the emotional labor of sensitive and feminist research methodologies. *Qualitative Research*, *13*(5), 546–561. doi:10.1177/1468794112455039.

Ceccarelli, L. (2001). Rhetorical criticism and the rhetoric of science. *Western Journal of Communication, 65*(3), 314–329. doi:10.1080/10570310109374708.

Ceccarelli, L. (2013). To whom do we speak? the audiences for scholarship on the rhetoric of science and technology. *Poroi, 9*(1) doi:10.13008/2151-2957.1151.

Charmaz, K., & Belgrave, L. L. (2015). Grounded theory. In G. Ritzer (Ed.), *The Blackwell Encyclopedia of Sociology* doi:10.1002/9781405165518.wbeosg 070.pub2.

Condit, C. (1984). The contemporary American abortion controversy: Stages in the argument. *Quarterly Journal of Speech, 70*(4), 410–424. doi:10.1080/0033 5638409383707.

Condit, C. M. (1990). *Decoding abortion rhetoric: Communicating social change.* Champaign, IL: University of Illinois Press.

Condit, C. M. (2013). "Mind the gaps": Hidden purposes and missing internationalism in scholarship on the rhetoric of science and technology in public discourse. *Poroi, 9*(1) doi:10.13008/2151-2957.1150.

Danisch, R. (2017). Rhetorical agency in a neoliberal age: Foucault, power, agency, and ethos. In K. H. Nguyen (Ed.), *Rhetoric in neoliberalism* (pp. 63–85). Cham: Palgrave Macmillan. Retrieved from https://link.springer.com/chapter/10.1007/ 978-3-319-39850-1_4

De Hertogh, L. B. (2015). Reinscribing a new normal: Pregnancy, disability, and health 2.0 in the online natural birthing community, birth without fear. *Ada: A Journal of Gender, New Media and Technology*, (7), n.p.

Dhai, A. (2017). Exploitation of the vulnerable in research: Responses to lessons learnt in history. *South African Medical Journal, 107*(6), 472–474. doi:10.7196/ SAMJ.2017.v107i6.12437.

Dolmage, J. (2009). Metis, Mêtis, Mestiza, Medusa: Rhetorical bodies across rhetorical traditions. *Rhetoric Review, 28*(1), 1–28. doi:10.1080/0735019080 2540690.

Dolmage, J. (2015). Universal design: Places to start. *Disability Studies Quarterly, 35*(2) doi:10.18061/dsq.v35i2.4632.

Dolmage, J. (2017). *Academic ableism: Disability and higher education.* Ann Arbor, MI: University of Michigan Press. Retrieved from https://muse.jhu.edu/book/ 57058

Dusenbery, M. (2018). *Doing harm: The truth about how bad medicine and lazy science leave women dismissed, misdiagnosed, and sick.* New York: Harper Collins.

Emmons, K. (2010). *Black dogs and blue words: Depression and gender in the age of self-care.* New Brunswick, NJ: Rutgers University Press.

Endres, D., Hess, A., Senda-Cook, S., & Middleton, M. K. (2016). In situ rhetoric. *Cultural Studies, Critical Methodologies, 16*(6), 511–524. doi:10.1177/153270 8616655820.

Fahnestock, J. (2005). Rhetoric of science: Enriching the discipline. *Technical Communication Quarterly, 14*(3), 277–286. doi:10.1207/s15427625tcq1403_5.

Fissell, M. E. (2006). *Vernacular bodies: The politics of reproduction in early modern England.* Oxford, UK: Oxford University Press.

Frances, A. (2012). Psychiatric mislabeling is bad for your mental health. *Psychology Today.* Retrieved from https://www.psychologytoday.com/za/blog/dsm5-in-distress/ 201205/psychiatric-mislabeling-is-bad-your-mental-health?amp

Francis, A. (2013). *Saving normal: An insider's revolt against out-of-control psychiatric diagnosis, DSM-5, big pharma, and the medicalization of ordinary life.* New York: Harper Collins.

Freddi, M. (2013). Developments and trends in the rhetoric of science: Science, rhetoric, culture. *European Journal of English Studies, 17*(3), 221–234. doi:10.1080/13825577.2013.867184.

Gibbons, M. G. (2014). Beliefs about the mind as doxastic inventional resource: Freud, neuroscience, and the case of Dr. Spock's baby and child care. *Rhetoric Society Quarterly, 44*(5), 427–448. doi:10.1080/02773945.2014.957411.

Gieryn, T. (1999). *Cultural boundaries of science.* Chicago, IL: University of Chicago Press.

Goldstein, D. (2015). Vernacular turns: Narrative, local knowledge, and the changed context of folklore. *The Journal of American Folklore, 128*(508), 125–145. doi:10.5406/jamerfolk.128.508.0125.

Graham, S. S. (2015). *The politics of pain medicine: A rhetorical-ontological inquiry.* Chicago, IL: University of Chicago Press.

Graham, S. S., & Herndl, C. (2013). Multiple ontologies in pain management: Toward a postplural rhetoric of science. *Technical Communication Quarterly, 22*(2), 103–125. doi:10.1080/10572252.2013.733674.

Gross, A. (1996). *The rhetoric of science.* Boston, MA: Harvard University Press.

Gross, A. (2008). Rhetoric of science. In W. Donsbach (Ed.), *The international encyclopedia of communication, first edition* (pp. 1–5). Hoboken, NJ: John Wiley & Sons, Ltd.

Harris, M. (2015). Three in the room. *Qualitative Health Research, 25*(12), 1689–1699. doi:10.1177/1049732314566324.

Hauser, G. A. (2011). Attending the vernacular: A plea for an ethnographical rhetoric. In C. Meyer & F. Girke (Eds.), *The rhetorical emergence of culture* (NED—New edition, 1 ed., pp. 157–172). New York: Berghahn Books.

Hauser, G. A., & McClellen, E. D. (2009). Vernacular rhetoric and social movements: Performances of resistance in the rhetoric of the everyday. In S. M. Stevens & P. M. Malesh (Eds.), *Active voices: Composing a rhetoric for social movements* (pp. 23–46). Albany, NY: State University of New York Press.

Heifferon, B. A. (2006). The new smallpox: An epidemic of words? *Rhetoric Review,* (1), 76.

Herndl, C. (2017). Introduction to the symposium on engaged rhetoric of science, technology, engineering and medicine. *Poroi, 12*(2) doi:10.13008/2151-2957.1259.

Herndl, C., & Cutlip, L. (2013). "How can we act?" A praxiographical program for the rhetoric of technology, science, and medicine. *Poroi, 9*(1) doi:10.13008/2151-2957.1163.

Hess, A. (2011). Critical-rhetorical ethnography: Rethinking the place and process of rhetoric. *Communication Studies, 62*(2), 127–152. doi:10.1080/10510974.2011.529750.

Holladay, D. (2017). Classified conversations: Psychiatry and tactical technical communication in online spaces. *Technical Communication Quarterly, 26*(1), 8–24. doi:10.1080/10572252.2016.1257744.

Hyde, M. (2014). *Ethos* and rhetoric. In W. Donsbach (Ed.), *The international encyclopedia of communication* (pp. 1604–1606). Hoboken, NJ: John R. Wylie

and Sons. Retrieved from https://onlinelibrary.wiley.com/doi/abs/10.1002/9781
405186407.wbiece043.pub2

Ingraham, C. (2013). Talking (about) the elite and mass: Vernacular rhetoric and discursive status. *Philosophy & Rhetoric, 46*(1), 1–21. doi:10.5325/philrhet. 46.1.0001.

Johnson, J. (2010). The skeleton on the couch: The Eagleton affair, rhetorical disability, and the stigma of mental illness. *Rhetoric Society Quarterly, 40*(5), 459–478. doi:10.1080/02773945.2010.517234.

Johnson, N. (2014). Enhancing the epistemological project in the rhetoric of science: Information infrastructure as tool for identifying epistemological commitments in scientific and technical communities. *Poroi, 10*(2). doi:10.13008/2151-2957. 1202.

Julian. (2016). Julian's story: "The stigma that still surrounds mental illness is remarkable." Retrieved from www.mentalhealth.org.uk/stories/julians-story-stigma-still-surrounds-mental-illness-remarkable

Jutel, A. G. (2011). *Putting a name to it: Diagnosis in contemporary society*. Baltimore, MD: Johns Hopkins University Press.

Kelly, P. A. (2014). Textual standardization and the DSM-5 "Common language." *Journal of Medical Humanities, 35*(2), 171–189. doi:10.1007/s10912-014-9281-9.

Keränen, L. (2010). *Scientific characters: Rhetoric, politics, and trust in breast cancer research*. Tuscaloosa: University of Alabama Press.

Keränen, L. (2014). This weird, incurable disease: Competing diagnoses in the rhetorics of Morgellons. In T. Jones, D. Wear, & L. Friedman (Eds.), *Health humanities reader* (pp. 36–51). New Brunswick: Rutgers University Press.

Kirsch, G. (2005). Friendship, friendliness, and feminist fieldwork. *Signs, 30*(4), 2163–2172. doi:10.1086/428415.

Koerber, A. L. (2013). *Breast or bottle?: Contemporary controversies in infant feeding policy and practice*. Columbia: University of South Carolina Press.

Kornelsen, J., Atkins, C., Brownell, K., & Woollard, R. (2016). The meaning of patient experiences of medically unexplained physical symptoms. *Qualitative Health Research, 26*(3), 367–376. doi:10.1177/1049732314566326.

Ladwig, K. H., Marten-Mittag, B., Erazo, N., & Gündel, H. (2001). Identifying somatization disorder in a population-based health examination survey: Psychosocial burden and gender differences. *Psychosomatics, 42*(6), 511–518. doi:10.1176/appi.psy.42.6.511.

Lewiecki-Wilson, C. (2003). Rethinking rhetoric through mental disabilities. *Rhetoric Review, 22*(2), 156–167.

Liehr, P., & Smith, M. J. (2017). Middle range theory: A perspective on development and use. *ANS. Advances in Nursing Science, 40*(1), 51–63. doi:10.1097/ANS.0000000000000162.

Mann, J. C. (2012). *Outlaw rhetoric: Figuring vernacular eloquence in Shakespeare's England*. Ithaca, NY: Cornell University Press.

McCarthy, L. P., & Gerring, J. P. (1994). Revising psychiatry's charter document: DSM-IV. *Written Communication, 11*(2), 147–192. doi:10.1177/0741088394 011002001.

Mcclellan, E. D. (2011). Narrative as vernacular rhetoric: Understanding community among transients, tourists and locals. *Storytelling, Self, Society, 7*(3), 188–210. doi:10.1080/15505340.2011.596089.

Melonçon, L., & Frost, E. A. (2015). Special issue introduction: Charting an emerging field: The rhetorics of health and medicine and its importance in communication design. *Communication Design Quarterly Review, 3*(4), 7–14. doi:10.1145/2826972.2826973.

Melonçon, L. K., & Scott, J. B. (2018a). Manifesting a scholarly dwelling place in RHM. *Rhetoric of Health & Medicine, 1*(1–2), x. doi:10.5744/rhm.2018.1001

Melonçon, L. K., & Scott, J. B. (2018b). *Methodologies for the rhetoric of health & medicine*. New York: Routledge.

Merton, R. K. (1968). *Social theory and social structure*. New York, NY: Simon and Schuster.

Miller, C. (2013). Audiences, brains, sustainable planets, and communication technologies: Four horizons for the rhetoric of science and technology. *Poroi, 9*(1). doi:10.13008/2151-2957.1159.

Molloy, C. (2015). Recuperative *ethos* and agile epistemologies: Toward a vernacular engagement with mental illness ontologies. *Rhetoric Society Quarterly, 45*(2), 138–163. doi:10.1080/02773945.2015.1010125.

Muckelbauer, J. (2016). Implicit paradigms of rhetoric: Aristotelian, cultural and heliotropic. In *Rhetoric through everyday things* (pp. 30–41). Tuscaloosa, AL: University of Alabama Press.

Ono, K. A., & Sloop, J. M. (1995). The critique of vernacular discourse. *Communication Monographs, 62*(1), 19–46. doi:10.1080/03637759509376346.

Opsal, T., Wolgemuth, J., Cross, J., Kaanta, T., Dickmann, E., Colomer, S., & Erdil-Moody, Z. (2016). "There are no known benefits . . . ": Considering the risk/benefit ratio of qualitative research. *Qualitative Health Research, 26*(8), 1137.

Owens, K. H. (2015). *Writing childbirth: Women's rhetorical agency in labor and online*. Carbondale, IL: SIU Press.

Parker, L. (2017, April 19). A letter to the doctor who didn't believe me. Retrieved from https://laraeparker.com/2017/04/18/a-letter-to-the-doctor-who-didnt-believe-me/

Perelman, C., & Olbrechts-Tyteca, L. (1971). *The new rhetoric: A treatise on argumentation*. Notre Dame: Notre Dame University Press. Retrieved from https://undpress.nd.edu/9780268004460/new-rhetoric-the

Phillips, J. D. (2012). Engaging men and boys in conversations about gender violence: Voice male magazine using vernacular rhetoric as social resistance. *The Journal of Men's Studies, 20*(3), 259–273. doi:10.3149/jms.2003.259.

Popham, S. L. (2014). Hybrid disciplinarity: Métis and *ethos* in juvenile mental health electronic records. *Journal of Technical Writing and Communication, 44*(3), 329–344. doi:10.2190/TW.44.3.f.

Porr, C., Drummond, J., & Olson, K. (2012). Establishing therapeutic relationships with vulnerable and potentially stigmatized clients. *Qualitative Health Research, 22*(3), 384–396. doi:10.1177/1049732311421182.

Prendergast, C. (2001). On the rhetoric of mental disability. In J. C. Wilson (Ed.), *Embodied rhetoric: Disability in language and culture* (pp. 47–60). Carbondale: Southern Illinois University Press.

Price, M. (2011). *Mad at school: Rhetorics of mental disability and academic life*. Lansing, MI: University of Michigan Press.

Reynolds, J. F. (2008). The rhetoric of mental health care. In B. Heifferon & S. C. Brown (Eds.), *Rhetoric of healthcare: Essays toward a new disciplinary inquiry* (pp. 149–157). Cresskill, NJ: Hampton Press.

Reynolds, J. F. (2018). A short history of mental health rhetoric research (MHRR). *Rhetoric of Health & Medicine, 1*(1–2), 1–18. doi:10.5744/rhm.2018.1003.

Reynolds, J. F., & Mair, D. C. (2013). *Writing and reading mental health records: Issues and analysis in professional writing and scientific rhetoric.* New York: Routledge. doi:10.4324/9780203811221.

Ringrose, J & Renold, E. (2014). *F**k rape!: Exploring affective intensities in a feminist research assemblage.* SAGE Publications Inc. doi:10.1177/1077800414530261.

Rothfelder, K., & Thornton, D. J. (2017). Man interrupted: Mental illness narrative as a rhetoric of proximity. *Rhetoric Society Quarterly, 47*(4), 359–382. doi: 10.1080/02773945.2017.1279343.

Schuster, M. L. (2006). A different place to birth: A material rhetoric analysis of baby haven, a free-standing birth center. *Women's Studies in Communication, 29*(1), 1–38. doi:10.1080/07491409.2006.10757626.

Scott, B. (2017, December). *Rhetoric in RHM* [video file]. Retrieved from https://www.youtube.com/watch?v=DA71IzviZBU

Scott, B., Segal, J., & Keränen, L. (2013). The rhetorics of health and medicine: Inventional possibilities for scholarship and engaged practice. *Poroi, 9*(1), 2–6. doi:10.13008/2151-2957.1157.

Segal, J., & Richardson, A. W. (2003). Introduction. scientific *ethos*: Authority, authorship, and trust in the sciences. *Configurations, 11*(2), 137–144. doi:10.1353/con.2004.0023.

Segal, J. Z. (2005). *Health and the rhetoric of medicine.* Carbondale, IL: Southern Illinois University Press.

Smith, C. M. (2010). Audiences and vernacular rhetoric. *Cultural Analysis, 9*, 65.

Spivak, G. C. (1988). Can the subaltern speak? In C. Nelson & L. Grossberg (Eds.), *Marxism and the interpretation of culture*) (pp. 271–313). Urbana, IL: University of Illinois Press.

St. Amant, K., & Graham, S. S. (2019). Research that resonates: A perspective on durable and portable approaches to scholarship in technical communication and rhetoric of science. *Technical Communication Quarterly, 28*(2), 99–111. doi:10.1080/10572252.2019.1591118.

Teston, C. (2017). *Bodies in flux: Scientific methods for negotiating medical uncertainty.* Chicago, IL: University of Chicago Press.

Thorvilson, M. J., & Copeland, A. J. (2018). Incompatible with care: Examining trisomy 18 medical discourse and families' counter-discourse for recuperative *ethos. The Journal of Medical Humanities, 39*(3), 349–360. doi:10.1007/s10912-017-9436-6.

Troup, C. L. (2009). Ordinary people can reason. *Journal of Business Ethics, 87*(4), 441–453.

Uthappa, N. R. (2017). Moving closer: Speakers with mental disabilities, deep disclosure, and agency through vulnerability. *Rhetoric Review, 36*(2), 164–175. doi:10.1080/07350198.2017.1282225.

van Delden, J. M, & van der Graaf, R. (2017). Revised CIOMS international ethical guidelines for health-related research involving humans. *Jama, 317*(2), 135–136. doi:10.1001/jama.2016.18977.

Vasquez, J. C., Fritz, G. K., Kopel, S. J., Seifer, R., McQuaid, E. L., & Canino, G. (2009). Ethnic differences in somatic symptom reporting in children with asthma and their parents. *Journal of the American Academy of Child & Adolescent Psychiatry, 48*(8), 855–863. doi:10.1097/CHI.0b013e3181a81333.

Vaughan-Williams, N., & Stevens, D. (2016). Vernacular theories of everyday (in)security: The disruptive potential of non-elite knowledge. *Security Dialogue, 47*(1), 40–58. doi:10.1177/0967010615604101.

Walsh, L. (2013). *Scientists as prophets: A rhetorical genealogy.* Oxford, NY: Oxford University Press.

Wells, S. (2010). *Our bodies, ourselves and the work of writing* | Palo Alto, CA: Stanford University Press.

White, W. (2014). Disciplinarity and the rhetoric of science: A social epistemological reception study. *Poroi, 10*(2) doi:10.13008/2151-2957.1130.

Zerbe, M. J. (2007). *Composition and the rhetoric of science: Engaging the dominant discourse.* Carbondale, IL: Southern Illinois University Press.

2 Vulnerable Rhetors and Stigma in Health and Medicine

Introduction

Notably, health and medical inequities[1] data "cluster around race, ethnicity, education, neighborhoods, and income" (Pereda & Montoya, 2018, p. 2), so the treatment patients receive in health and medical care settings can depend on demographics. Thus, basic material conditions (i.e., income level, insurance coverage, geographic location), account for some inequalities. Indeed, having more money, better insurance, higher education, and access to premier health and wellness institutions arguably makes better health outcomes much more likely. Some of these discrepancies, however, are due to care providers' beliefs about the veracity of patients' subjective reports of symptoms[2] and attendant misdiagnoses.

In some cases, then, a provider simply does not find the patient to be credible, and makes clinical judgments accordingly. This chapter continues to argue that rhetorical *ethos* (or credibility) is a particularly relevant framing mechanism for interrogating the roles stigmas and abuses play in patterns of persuasion as they relate to social reproduction. It accomplishes this goal by outlining what is known about the most pervasive, specific forms of stigmas and biases patients must contend with in their day-to-day lives. This deep dive into what is known about health inequities that I argue are related to assumed lack of credibility helps to carve out space for a better appreciation of the vernacular strategies participants develop, which are showcased in chapters to come. These strategies include, for example, assigning a credibility proxy (or having someone vouch for your reliability when you are unfairly doubted), and using appeals to recuperative *ethos* (or everyday appeals to credibility that are linked to contesting specific forms of intractable stigma).

As Chapter 1 demonstrated, rhetoric of health and medicine (RHM) and related scholarly movements carve out space for research grounded in vernacular rhetorical theories with a specific emphasis on *ethos*. Such inquiries might lead to important insights into how patients can advocate for best care since health conditions unfold in the context of everyday life and seeking care for health conditions involves a good amount of dense persuasion on both sides of the exam table. Chapter 1 specifically uses RHM-related scholarship alongside vernacular rhetorical work to build a case for exploring rhetorical *ethos* and its ongoing role in recovering the physical, social, emotional, and professional losses that come with unjust or stigmatizing health and medical experiences. Chapters 3, 4, and 5 offer specific cases of patient strategies for building and rebuilding strong *ethos* in their pursuits of better care and more livable lives. This chapter does the important work of paving the way for the work to come by synthesizing what is known about biases, stigmas, and inadequate care.

Intersectional Marks of Difference, Anchoring Bias, and Psychogenic Diagnosis

The ways that intersectional marks of difference make an impact on clinical exchanges (and in the diagnostic process and beyond) are well documented in sociological and medical anthropological literature as well as in interdisciplinary health sciences literature. Specifically, this scholarship demonstrates that overlapping markers of gender, race, and social class impact doctor-patient relations and lead to inadequate care, to misdiagnoses of psychogenic symptoms, and to more diagnoses of mental health problems in general. Just as well, cultural factors impact clinical exchanges (Alarcón, 2009; Cockerham, 2016; Jutel, 2010; Munch, 2004; St. Amant, 2017; Schwartz & Blankenship, 2014). This literature, when discussing health outcomes for diverse patient groups, is careful to distinguish between noted differences that are perhaps not bias-related versus those that are true inequities. Williams and colleagues (2015) eloquently argued that "disparities in health and health care" are pervasive and that "extensive evidence shows differences across racial/ethnic, gender, and geographic groupings" (p. 758). They also showed that "access to health care, cultural and language differences, communication and trust barriers, and socioeconomic differences are clearly contributors to these disparities" and, importantly, that "stereotyping or decisional biases by clinicians in some situations may also play a role" (Williams et al., 2015, p. 758). That said, even health outcomes that are not directly attributable to bias likely have their roots in insidious, difficult-to-trace, systemic forms of inequality.

Biases, of course, impact "decision making, resulting in medical errors and negative patient outcomes" (Busby, Courtier, & Glastonbury, 2018, p. 246). Indeed, once a care provider makes a decision about a person's credibility, it is very difficult for the patient to alter the provider's perceptions. This is a major problem because a provider's belief that a patient is unreliable could mean missed opportunities for appropriate care. For example, among the many biases that Busby et al. (2018) identified is the well-known "anchoring bias," or "a situation in which a person remains firm in their initial diagnostic impression, despite being presented with additional subsequent contrary information" (p. 237). Forms of bias, including anchoring bias, are interconnected. They overlap and interweave themselves into complex configurations of cause and effect. Thus, anchoring biases can have origins in racial/ethnic, gender, and/or socioeconomic status judgments or some mix of these. In all cases, anchoring biases are dangerous, as they often lead to misdiagnosis. That said, there is likely rarely ill will on the part of the provider.

As Chapter 3 will show, many anchoring biases take the form of inaccurate psychogenic diagnoses. One participant, for example, described how she'd been diagnosed with anxiety and depression for over a decade despite repeated clinical visits with new and worsening symptoms. When her symptoms did not respond to antidepressants and therapy, doctors doubled down treatment efforts aimed at anxiety and depression. It was only after she tried the Paleo diet, famous for being grain-free, that she noticed her symptoms disappear nearly overnight. Readers, this was after over ten years of repeated, frustrating, and costly medical appointments where she was repeatedly told that her symptoms were "all in her head," and she needed to try harder to be well by fixing her mental health via being a compliant mental health patient.

After doing her own research following her Paleo diet experience, she concluded that she likely had celiac disease. The patient asked her physician to do a simple blood test, and, finally, she had an accurate diagnosis. However, the years she spent on antidepressants she didn't need and the years she spent inflaming her small intestine with gluten caused long-term damage. If a simple blood test would have been given early on or at any point in her journey prior to her self-diagnosis, she would have avoided some chronic consequences, not least of which is a complete distrust of medical professionals.

Undoubtedly, the fact that she was a young woman when she sought care and follow-up care led to anchoring bias. *Doxa* or popular opinion very much supports the idea that young women are prone to depression and anxiety. This misconception has origins in a number of popular-culture texts. Care providers determined that she had both conditions. No new evidence could convince them otherwise until her own bodily experiments, what Kalin and Gruber (2018) would call skilled "experimentation," (p. 286) led to a total reversal of symptoms. As a result of such factors, an anchoring bias in favor of a psychological explanation for symptoms prevented a more expedient diagnosis of a physical disease. It is likely that this participants' provider could not see past the depressed/anxious diagnosis to consider other potential causes. Cases such as this illustrate the complexity of credibility and its impact on care.

Care Providers' Awareness of Credibility's Impact on Care

Physicians themselves are not blind to the impact of credibility on care, of course. Most do not set out to do harm, and some devote their research and writing efforts to related causes. In a recent *Washington Post* article, for example, Bhargava (2019) used her clinical experience with lung cancer patients to express a deep concern with stigma and its relation to blaming patients for their conditions. She noted that "the tight link between tobacco and lung cancer has hardened into stigma, and the potential for care disparities is real" (n.p.). Bhargava emphasized that "our culture's tendency to frame certain illnesses as character defects, as opposed to complex phenomena with genetic and psychosocial components, is widespread and carries serious consequences" (n.p.).

Bhargava's (2019) piece makes it clear that the quality and tenor of treatment can be adversely altered when care providers do not find their patients to be sympathetic consumers of healthcare services or even worthwhile human persons. In fact, when physicians believe character flaws or poor lifestyle choices lead to disease, *kakoethos* or "bad character," comes into play. This misinformation on patients' credibility is "both rhetorically constituted and rhetorically disabling" (Johnson, 2010, p. 460). Assuming patients' symptoms are "all in their heads," or considering a patient too "mentally ill" to accurately convey physical and mental symptoms, can do just as much damage and follows the same impulse. In both cases, the speaker/patient is not considered a credible source of useful clinical information on verifiable physical diseases. The assumption may even be that the things a patient says are always already signs of psychosis. Taking these realities together, it is quite possible that a care providers' inaccurate beliefs about a person's credibility can, in the worst cases, render them especially vulnerable to preventable morbidity and even mortality.

Implicit Bias, Cognitive Bias, and *Ethos*

When a physician makes a diagnostic judgment call about a patient, it is inevitably tied up not only in self-reported symptoms and clinical observations, but also in the assessment of the person's credibility. Importantly, care providers do not consciously hold biased views toward their patients, but often carry, instead, what researchers have called "implicit bias"[3] (Teachman & Brownell, 2001), or "an unintentional, unacknowledged preference for one group over another" (Chapman, Kaatz, & Carnes, 2013, p. 1508). It should be noted that "implicit bias occurs without conscious awareness and is frequently at odds with one's personal beliefs" (Chapman et al., 2013, p. 1504). That is, implicit bias does not indicate widespread, overt biases in physicians, but signals, instead, disparities between self-reported inclusive ideologies and everyday clinical behaviors. This relationship can be seen in, for example, instances where a highly educated, compassionate, inclusive provider without any stated biases unconsciously judges a patient's self-reported symptoms based on stereotypes. Similarly, cognitive biases—systematic and often unconscious substitutions of socially constructed attitudes for objective facts—"influence diagnostic accuracy, management, and therapeutic decisions" (Saposnik, Redelmeier, Ruff, & Tobler, 2016, p. 12).

Evidence that attests to the inconsistencies of clinical judgment are not new. As the previous section argued, medical professionals themselves are well aware of the vagaries of their day-to-day work and of the capacity for human error—even in the context of very good intentions; as Schuman (2017) powerfully put it:

> We in the medical profession pride ourselves on the ideal of treating all patients, regardless of color, creed, gender, sexuality, legal, financial or health status. Sadly, we often fall far short, subject to our own biases and preconceptions about people based on how they look or, especially, how they interact with us.
>
> (n.p.)

Clearly, "disparities linger and may lead to unacceptable increases in morbidity and mortality for some," and "implicit bias, an unintentional, unacknowledged preference for one group over another" is one key area of concern (Chapman et al., 2013, p. 1508). Research supports, then, that patient care is impacted by physician biases (Chapman et al., 2013, p. 1507), and, predictably, implicit racism plays an especially troubling role in healthcare disparities.

The Institute of Medicine's *Unequal treatment* report on racial and ethnic disparities in healthcare (Smedley, Stith & Nelson, 2003), in fact, emphasized that while socioeconomic status impacted health outcomes, race was perhaps even more of an issue. The report found that even with controls for socioeconomic differences, care providers held more stereotypes of black patients. For example, care providers considered low socioeconomic status black patients "less pleasant and less rational" than low socioeconomic status white patients (p. 166). This is not, of course, to lessen the importance of socioeconomic factors, but to emphasize that the role racism plays in care settings is even more problematic.

Emphasizing cross-cultural training to improve patient-provider communication, the report inspired a wealth of research into the topic of medical disparities based in racial biases. Relatedly, Druckman and colleagues' (2018) vignette study of college athletes and pain reinforced previous findings, "showing a racial bias in pain perception whereby people . . . assume blacks feel less pain than do whites" (p. 727). Medical students and residents also exhibit "racial bias in pain assessment and treatment recommendations" rooted in "beliefs about biological differences between blacks and whites—beliefs dating back to slavery—associated with the perception that black people feel less pain than do white people" (Hoffman, Trawalter, Axt, & Oliver, 2016, p. 4300).

Among disparities that rest on racial lines, "suboptimal pain care is common, especially for black patients," and while "several factors contribute to this disparity," one important factor is "provider biases" (Hirsh, Hollingshead, Ashburn-Nardo, & Kroenke, 2015, p. 2).

Finding significant racial disparities in two of 18 sites where abusive head trauma is treated, Hymel et al. (2018), likewise, noted that "local provider implicit bias" (p. 141) has a relationship to race-based inequities. Cuevas, O'Brien, and Saha (2017) also found that "disparities in the quality of clinician-patient relationships arise from ethnic minority patients being treated differently than European American patients" and that "in general, patients have similar preferences but receive unequal treatment" (p. 8).

Importantly, "the conditions predicting when implicit biases will predict behavior or not are not yet fully understood" as there can be a "lack of a significant correlation" between providers' implicit and explicit biases (Oliver, Wells, Joy-Gaba, Hawkins & Nosek, 2014, p. 183).

As Oliver et al. (2014) succinctly put it, "studies of the possible role of implicit racial biases on clinical decision making should continue, and tools should be developed to help clinicians mitigate the effect of such biases on clinical practice" (p. 185). Hymel and colleagues (2018) also indicated that "practice disparities and implicit bias" are best addressed by "evidence-based" rules and regulations (p. 142). Many of these tools or remedies for racial disparities in healthcare are explored in the literature, including "critical dialogue" on race, which might mitigate the "difficult and uncomfortable" nature of open dialogues on race by "normalizing the process of accepting responsibility and learning how to rectify errors that may occur" (Tsai et al., 2018, p. 694).

Interestingly, despite the data supporting racial bias as more prevalent than socioeconomic status bias, these findings are inconsistent. Druckman and colleagues' (2018) study of student athletes showed that racial bias was "mediated by socioeconomic status" (p. 727). Specifically, they found that the assumption that black people feel less pain correlated to the belief that persons of color have lower socioeconomic status, leading the researchers to recommend "interventions grounded in recognizing that social class and the hardship it conveys do not make one impervious to physical pain" (Druckman et al., 2018, p. 728). And, while some studies point to race as the most pressing area of concern in terms of health-outcome disparities based in biases, others indicate that socioeconomic status is more of an issue. Some studies demonstrate "the existence of both racial and socioeconomic health disparity," but also find that "socioeconomic status" has "the most substantial impact on health disparity" (Bowman et al., 2010, p. 778). Dougall and Schwartz (2011) found similar socioeconomic status bias in psychotherapy where they noted that "cognitive reactions can impact [care providers'] clinical judgments" (n.p.).

In their study of medical students, Pettit and colleagues (2017) found that they touched lower socioeconomic status (SES) patients more frequently than higher socioeconomic patients, but asked higher socioeconomic patients about pain control more often. The authors attributed the additional touching to medical students wishing to demonstrate empathy (p. 129). However, they also noted that the behavior difference correlated to power dynamics, with a doctor's more frequent touching meant as a power move (p. 129). Likewise, while Williams et al. (2015) did not find racial bias in their study of clinical encounters, they "did find a clear variation in student recommendations by patient SES, with the highest SES patients more likely to receive procedural recommendations" (p. 763).

Accounting for Inconsistencies in Research on Biases in Healthcare

At times, too, studies find no correlation between implicit biases and clinical decision-making, but researchers are careful to point out that these findings are not entirely reliable and that implicit biases do negatively impact clinical outcomes. In addition to mixed results on the predominance of race-based and socioeconomic-status-based biases, the literature on the existence of bias is inconsistent. Due to variations in methodological rigor and scope of studies, many of which are focus groups, computer-simulated patients, vignette survey studies, or non-observational studies, some find no empirical evidence of bias at all. Interestingly, Haider and colleagues (2011) used their data from vignette-based clinical assessments with medical students to indicate that while biases based on race and social class exist, they do not necessarily impact clinical decision-making. Other studies, though, are quite clear on the implications of biases for clinical outcomes. These studies emphasize that *perception* is the issue rather than actually problematic practices; for example, Cuevas et al. (2017) found that "while preferences for care were mostly similar across groups, experiences differed in ways that patients, particularly African American patients, perceived as discriminatory" (p. 9). Haider and colleagues (2015) found that a "high prevalence of implicit biases among RNs did not translate to a proxy of the nurses' provision of care" (p. 1084). They also noted that the "presence of an unconscious bias was not associated with any overall differences in vignette-based clinical assessment and decision making by nurse providers" (Haider et al., 2015, p. 1084).

However, authors are clear that they do not take their findings to mean that biases and attendant medical error in clinical encounters do not exist. Instead, astute authors conclude that systematically studying the impact of bias on clinical decision-making is exceedingly difficult work and is not always adequately measured "in a simulation environment" (Pettit et al., 2017, p. 129). They note that participants are often aware of (or guess at) the nature of the studies in which they are involved, so their behaviors could be altered as a result. On the topic of their study of clinicians from surgical and other related specialties, Haider, Schneider, Sriram, Scott et al. (2015) found that data "did not demonstrate any association between implicit race or social class bias and clinical decision making" (p. 462). That said, the authors also noted that "existing biases might influence the quality of care received by minority patients and those of lower socioeconomic status in real-life clinical encounters" (p. 462). Researchers, thus, share the inclinations that simulations-based studies might not accurately measure the potentially problematic impact of biases on actual clinical encounters.

Maina, Belton, Ginzberg, Singh, and Johnson's (2018) review of literature on clinical biases found that there is a "growing body of literature" to suggest that care providers "across multiple levels of training and disciplines" hold racial biases (p. 224). They also found that, predictably, care providers of color are less likely to exhibit such biases. Still, the authors point out that there is "limited research examining the impact of implicit bias on patient care and outcomes," and that "most studies have been vignette-based and reveal mixed results," with only four providing concrete evidence of implicit bias and eight finding no correlation (p. 224). However, the authors are clear that there is a known association "between higher implicit bias and poorer patient-provider interactions" and, notably, of the two studies that look at specific interventions and their outcomes, "only one has demonstrated postintervention reduction in implicit bias" (p. 224).

Thus, more research is necessary on which interventions might best address bias in clinical encounters.

The use of rhetorical *ethos* as a theoretical frame makes it possible to imagine how implicit biases impact clinical encounters in a very specific way. In Chapter 3, therefore, I share data from an interview study wherein I asked participants to share their strategies for establishing their credibility in clinical encounters when their doctors have doubted their symptoms or dismissed their complaints as "in their heads," and that focus led to verbatim reiterations of clinical conversations from a very specific vantage point that privileges the patients' experiences. In Chapter 5, moreover, I share ethnographic observations conducted at a community care facility for adults with chronic mental illnesses and examine their everyday exchanges through the lens of rhetorical *ethos*. Through a focus on how and why certain demographic markers might meld with discursive behaviors in real time to render a specific patient, in the care provider's estimation, less than credible, I hope to add to the literature on biases in health and medical care by showing how patients successfully push back against such underestimations of their worth in their everyday encounters with healthcare professionals and beyond. After all, these unconscious biases in clinical care, in favor of or against certain patients, infiltrate everyday life beyond the clinic, and they are chartable, in part, as issues of rhetorical *ethos*. A look at women's specific experiences in care settings reinforces the notion that credibility can negatively impact clinical encounters.

Women's Pain, Mental Health, and Misdiagnosis

On an otherwise ordinary Wednesday, journalist Fassler (2015) brought his partner to their local emergency department as she was experiencing debilitating abdominal pain. There, she endured hours of being patronized, dismissed, and misdiagnosed. In fact, she was given inappropriate treatment for kidney stones that she did not have and was told that her pain could not be as bad as she was reporting. After a young female doctor's[4] shift began many hours later and after Fassler vociferously advocated for his partner,[5] an accurate diagnosis of a much more serious condition was rendered: ovarian torsion—an excruciating and life-threatening medical emergency. Fassler was moved to write about the infantilizing, unkind treatment his ordinarily unflappable wife received. Focusing on the near-death nature of the sequence of events and the long-term impact of the experience, he noted that "she's still grappling with the psychic toll—what she calls 'the trauma of not being seen'" (n.p.).

While Fassler's essay registers his shock and disappointment with such poor initial care, those who've been similarly summarily dismissed in care settings likely do not find the narrative all that surprising, if still unsettling. Those familiar with the literature on gender discrimination in health and medicine, likewise, might not find the young female doctor's ability to treat the actual medical problem—missed by her older male colleague—surprising, either. As noted above, one major area of concern in terms of patient credibility, then, is whether or not pain is taken seriously as a sign of disease, as the literature demonstrates that racial and socioeconomic class-based discriminations can play a role in care providers' perceptions of pain. Likewise, "women who seek help are less likely than men to be taken seriously when they report pain and are less likely to have their pain adequately treated" (Hoffman & Tarzian, 2001, p. 19).

In recent years, the topic of women's pain, its relation to assumed mental health issues, and whether or not it is believable or believed has become a topic not only in popular journalism, but also in social media conversations thanks, in part, to celebrities' public statements on their fraught paths to treatment for difficult-to-diagnose and -treat conditions. For example, author and actress Dunham (2018), whose credibility is often called into question, made her decision to have a hysterectomy public via Instagram and magazine articles. Dauntingly, Dunham explained, doctors doubted her endometrial pain, favored psychological explanations for her symptoms, and indicated that they were more committed to maintaining her fertility than to ending her discomfort. Making matters worse, her exchanges with care providers left her feeling unable to grapple with the loss of her uterus. As she put it in a *Vogue* essay, "Because I had to work so hard to have my pain acknowledged, there was no time to feel fear or grief. To say goodbye. I made a choice that never was a choice for me, yet mourning feels like a luxury I don't have" (n.p.). Likewise, singer and actress Lady Gaga has shared her struggles with the contested and little-understood condition fibromyalgia on Twitter and elsewhere (Spector, 2017). As she put her experiences in a Twitter post:

> Before I was diagnosed, my own doctor brushed off my reports of pain and exhaustion for months, warning me to "trust the team" at the office and quit Googling. An allergist asked me with a leering smirk if I was "an allergic little girl," and then, after examining me and looking over my by-now encyclopedic folder of medical tests, said: "You're clearly very healthy."
>
> (Lady Gaga, 2017, as cited in Vincent, 2017, n.p.).

Journalist Weiss's (2018) Twitter post similarly asked:

> Women with chronic illnesses: how long & how many doctors did it take you to get diagnosed? I counted 11 months & 17 doctors & wrote down what each did to show what we go through just to begin to heal.
>
> (n.p.)

Weiss's initial tweet garnered 429 retweets, 390 comments, and 975 likes. Women from all walks of life responded and engaged with Weiss's post to share their own stories of misdiagnoses that they believe stem from sexism.[6] These women writers' assessments of their experiences are supported in the literature on gender discrimination and delayed or inaccurate medical diagnosis as researchers are able to confirm patterns of "separation between men and women, not embedded in biological differences but gendered norms" (Samulowitz, Gremyr, Eriksson, & Hensing, 2018, p. 9).

Importantly, though, much like racial and social class biases, research has shown that gender discrimination is often implicit. As such, the attributions of negative stereotypes to a patient by virtue of their gender is unconscious, and "additional research is," thus, "needed to better understand why women and men may receive different care when they have similar clinical characteristics (Daugherty et al., 2017, p. 9). As noted above, biases in care settings can be particularly difficult to trace and address since physicians are not necessarily cognizant of the biases or their influence on clinical decision-making. Samulowitz et al. (2018), thus, noted that "awareness about gendered norms" is necessary "both in research and clinical practice, in order to counteract gender bias in health care and to support health-care professionals in providing more equitable care" (p. 11). Relatedly, researchers have turned their attention to women's risk factors for cardiovascular disease and to the realities of women misunderstanding those risks (Kentner & Grace, 2017, p. 22). Such work highlights disparities in clinical research and its dissemination.

Much like the literature on biases based in race and socioeconomic status, then, the scholarship on gender-based biases in clinical encounters clearly points to the need for more research from a variety of perspectives, as permeating the thick sociocultural web of disparities in healthcare settings is highly complex work. It is also worth noting that much more research needs to be done to unpack the impact of intersectional marks of difference on credibility in clinical encounters. Indeed, the unique experiences of minority women, socioeconomically disadvantaged women, and trans women in care settings deserves much more attention. After all, it would stand to reason that more marks of difference can multiply the likelihood of being mistrusted in clinical exchanges and beyond, even as access and quality of care due to material realties join up with forces like implicit bias. Matters of credibility in these contexts can be, quite simply, matters of life and death. When care providers find patients to lack credibility,[7] inappropriate or even life-threatening care decisions are real risks. Moreover, the fraught dividing line between physical and mental health problems showcases the need for more critical explorations of this binary and for more sensitive appreciations of the permeable boundaries between bodies and minds. This inquiry highlights the fact that bodies and minds are not quite as separable as they would seem to be in how patients receive care. In relation to psychological diagnoses, too, such factors as implicit and cognitive bias can become exceedingly complex since mental health problems (or even the assumption of their existence) incite an incredible amount of distrust and stigma.

Mental Illness Diagnoses and Stigma

Mental health diagnoses provoke incredibly recalcitrant stigma (Hinshaw, 2006), and this stigma is often used as a way to discredit rhetors with nonstandard methods of seeing and living in the world. Since mental health diagnoses can damage credibility, fear of being labelled mentally ill, as Masterson (2018) made clear, can also lead to avoiding treatment. Due to the severely disabling nature of mental illness stigma in particular, several online activist spaces and initiatives exist in response to stigma. Many of these schemes include invitations for those who've experienced stigma to tell their stories. Sharing their experiences is meant to bring awareness to issues of discrimination. One example is the "See Me Social Movement,"[8] a Glasgow-based activist site where personal stories are shared in efforts to advance equal rights. As one woman, identified only as Susan, explained on that site: "Due to the stigma around mental illness I find there are times when I'm not taken seriously when I make suggestions. This has happened particularly at work. People will dismiss what I say and say, 'oh she is just reacting like that because of her illness'" (n.p.).

Susan's story astutely summarizes the credibility issues that often follow a mental health diagnosis. It is not difficult to imagine that other marks of difference only exacerbate those issues. As well, her story illustrates the way that "medical (especially mental illness) diagnoses" can be used as tools "for silencing others, neutralizing counterclaims, depoliticizing debate, or pre-empting it altogether." This problem is exacerbated with "a growing range of mental illness labels available" (Adorjan, Christensen, Kelly, & Pawluch, 2012, p. 469). These labels can be unjustly "used by social actors against those with different experiences, views, beliefs, and ideologies" (Adorjan et al., 2012, p. 469). In other words, Susan's colleagues might, at times, doubt her because they find her less credible since she has a mental health diagnosis. They might also unconsciously or consciously exploit her diagnosis in power moves when they simply do not agree with her stances. Having the opportunity to tell her story gives her space to show meta-awareness of the inequities at play when her diagnosis is used to dismiss her in the workplace. That said, there is little evidence to suggest that telling her story actually changes her coworkers' inappropriate behaviors toward her. In fact, unfortunately, anti-stigma campaigns have not yet been a match for the obstinacy of mental illness stigmas. This daunting reality makes the need for on-the-spot, everyday *ethos*-building and -rebuilding strategies necessary additions to stigmatized persons' vernacular arsenals. This book argues that such repositories of social energies can be extrapolated from everyday data.

Stigma's Staying Power

Despite the positive energy devoted to this and related disclosures-based anti-stigma efforts, Pescosolido et al. (2010) showed that well-meaning movements to end stigma often fail. For example, the push in the 1990s to equate mental illnesses with other, less stigmatizing health conditions by showcasing mental health problems as neurological ones technically succeeded. More people in the 2000s accepted the idea that mental illnesses were not moral failings, but brain diseases. However, this shift in understanding did not change the general public's unwillingness to accept those with mental illnesses into their communities. Participants indicated that they did not want to live near or work closely with someone with mental health problems, nor have a person with such problems marry into their families (p. 6). Pescosolido, Medina, Martin, & Long (2013) more recently noted that stigma is a global issue; they emphasized, though, that localized, "novel messages and approaches" are needed to address "the penetrating and damaging nature of prejudice" (p. 859). Their work highlighted the fact that stigma:

- originates in social relations
- is diffuse in everyday life, and
- is extremely difficult to combat.

Once a person is deemed "mentally ill," they are often no longer considered "rhetorically enabled subjects" (Prendergast, 2001, p. 56). That is to say that they are assumed to have no real contributions to make to public discourse, and any attempts they do make to participate in these or even private deliberations are treated as highly unreliable. This daunting portrait of stigma's staying power around the globe brings into sharp focus the issues and problems that arise in health and medical contexts when credibility is doubted. An examination of somatic symptom diagnoses similarly highlights the role of rhetorical *ethos* (i.e., credibility) in health and medical contexts.

How Biases Complicate Somatic Symptoms Diagnoses

Of course, all forms of bias can lead to higher instances of diagnoses of physical symptoms that are "in the patient's head," as the notion that bodily suffering has no real organic etiology is, of course, a mental illness known colloquially as hypochondria and subsumed in the most recent version of the DSM-V as "somatic symptom and related disorder"[9] (APA, 2013). That is, as the literature cited above makes clear, if a care provider deems the speaker less than credible, they are more likely to distrust the severity or even reality of physical symptoms. The belief, of course, that the patient's subjective symptoms report is a sign of mental health problems exacerbates other problems with rhetorical *ethos* that the patient must contend with. Indeed, "pain that is not readily explained medically has frequently been attributed to psychopathology," explained Katz, Rosenbloom, and Fashler (2015), and "the misdiagnosis of medical illness as mental illness" is a real risk (2015, p. 165).

Interestingly, explained Henningsen (2016), symptoms that are deemed "all in the patient's head" are not entirely unreliable; many of these diagnoses can be accurate or even helpful. However, that accuracy is severely compromised when diagnostic tests are not used to determine whether or not some physical cause is to blame for the symptoms; thus, "rational and systematic diagnostic testing" must be used to rule out organic causes for physicians to confidently and competently render a somatic symptoms diagnosis and attendant therapeutic measures (2016, p. 59). Care providers must be mindful of "the high probability of misdiagnosing a medical illness, including chronic pain conditions, as a mental illness" (Katz et al., 2015, p. 164).

Clearly, the data on stigma and bias in care settings, when considered alongside the work on misdiagnosis of somatic symptom and related disorders, indicates that more research is needed from various fronts on these important topics. As Chapter 1 makes clear, this book aims to take part in the scholarly tradition of showcasing the benefits of hybrid approaches to rhetoric scholarship in general (and the affordances of rhetorical *ethos* as a framing mechanism in particular) for building generative theories. Sociological, medical, and anthropological studies offer rich empirical data to support the ideas that mental health problems are stigmatizing; that race, class, and gender impact care decisions; and that psychogenic diagnoses are often inaccurate. Rhetorical frameworks offer insights into ways that *individuals* can use rhetorical tactics to build the kind of credibility that can push back against stigma and that might even help to mitigate the potential for a misdiagnosis of psychogenic symptoms and/or to minimize the social and emotional impact of a mental illness diagnosis.

Online Testaments to Misdiagnosis and Stigma

Everyday narrative accounts of postponed diagnoses and misdiagnoses of psychological problems in the medically ill abound online, and such discursive spaces highlight the complex interplay between health—both physical and mental—and gender, race, and socioeconomic class as these relate to credibility. The site *The Mighty: We Face Disease, Disability and Mental Illness Together*, "a digital health community created to empower and connect people facing health challenges and disabilities," is a particularly strong example ("The Mighty," n.p.). On this site, diverse writers share their stories of being discriminated against due to race and gender and to being doubted, misdiagnosed, and prescribed inappropriate courses of treatment for mental health issues from which they do not happen to suffer. Some writers lament the loss of social standing that came with their mental health diagnoses due to stigma, and others share their day-to-day struggles with chronic conditions.

In a compelling recent post, Masterson (2018), a PhD in health psychology and behavioral medicine, discussed her fears of becoming labelled "the worried well," or a healthy patient who is a frequent consumer of unnecessary health and medical appointments and attendant costly diagnostic tests. Her desire to avoid this label in her medical charts to maintain her credibility as a "sane" person led her to ignore symptoms of Sjögren's Syndrome for over a decade.[10]

Another writer described her desire to fulfill her dreams of becoming an academic while struggling with schizoaffective disorder and the lack of appropriate accommodations—another consequence of stigma. She explained: "I am determined to reach the top of academia, diagnosis in tow. It may take me longer than usual and I may need to have continued support and help, but I will get there. This illness is not going to get the better of me" (Rowe, 2018, n.p.). This writer draws on the common trope of dissociating from a diagnostic label by describing a condition as an external enemy with which the individual—a separate and separable agent—must fight. Rather than framing the need for accommodations as a reasonable expectation in an academic program, the writer is clear that the "support and help" will be considered excessive and will be hard won. Such discourses, ironically, reify inadequate accommodations, as they indicate that a strong and worthy opponent of a condition will win her fight, which will be clear when she is able to go about things in a "normal" way after successfully pleading for extraordinary assistance.

Another writer, Krys Clark (2018), described how her nine-month-old son was mistreated in an emergency room (ER) because he is black. After recounting how the ER's negligence nearly led to his death, she asserted:

> I know what I experienced earlier that day in the ER with my son was more than inadequate care. The doctor was curt, dismissive and her implicit racial bias influenced her decision to prematurely discharge my son. It could have killed him.
>
> (n.p.)

Online narratives from everyday web authors on sites like *The Mighty* confirm what many of us know to be true anecdotally, from personal experiences, or from informal conversations. In everyday life, indelible demographic markers hit up against social performances in health and medical (or medicalized) spaces to create on-the-spot *ethos* or credibility. *Ethos* is, thus, a powerful lens through which to illuminate inequities in diagnostics and treatment protocols as well as in everyday life. Rhetorical *ethos*-building and -rebuilding is especially necessary, I argue, in the context of particularly formidable stigmas and biases as they are described in this chapter.

Conclusion

When examining forms of bias as they impact medical decisions, one might ask: When life and death are on the line, is that the time to be fighting the patriarchy, the one percent, the heteronormative and transphobic? Yes and no. Vernacular exchanges can plant seeds of rebellion. Sophistry, in its most positive and generative sense, is alive and well in the participants I had the pleasure of observing, as well as the interview participants I spoke with on their savvy ways of arguing for their credibility when it is doubted in care settings. The following chapters share, in modest form, the ways that everyday rhetors push back against stigma that could be misread as unremarkable. Collected, parsed, and analyzed via rhetorical *ethos*, their efficacy becomes clearer.

Through a deeper look at stigmas and biases in health and medical contexts, this chapter continues the project of showcasing the value of rhetorically focused humanities projects for unpacking especially thorny health and medical realities by taking up a "rhetorical approach to illness and disease" as these approaches "call attention to the role of language in shaping meaning and action" (Keränen, 2014, p. 48). The literature cited above makes clear that a care provider's beliefs about a person are impacted by demographic features that exceed the clinical scene just as much as their beliefs are impacted in the real-time interactions that happen in the context of a medical appointment. Rhetorical *ethos*, in its generative analytic power, is naturally a part of health and medical realities in myriad ways as *ethos* as a rhetorical mechanism gives way to critical questions such as: Who is believed? Who is believable? In what contexts? And most importantly for this book: Why are some people believed while others are not? What can speakers do to render themselves more believable?

Significantly, this book does not offer readers ways for patients to lie to doctors so that they can get diagnostic tests or diagnoses that are inappropriate. Instead, the focus is on offering theoretical frameworks through which to conceptualize how some rhetorical moves render a person's *ethos* stronger such that they are able to tell their truths of body and mind and have them believed—particularly in instances in which stigmas and stereotypes alter the dialogic scene and lead to missed signs of disease or, quite the opposite, the appearance of mental illness where none is present. Likewise, this book aims to destigmatize mental health conditions by dispelling common myths to allow for more individuals' fuller participation in aspects of community life that are easy to take for granted, including worthwhile employment, nurturing relationships, and material stability. As a way to make space for the data and emergent theories to follow, this chapter has sought to further highlight the role a person's credibility can play in the care they receive and in the treatment (medical and otherwise) they get in everyday life. It does so by sharing ways that gender, race, and socioeconomic class alongside mental health stigmas and assumed psychogenic symptoms function to lessen credibility and to create conditions in which everyday *ethos*-building and -rebuilding tactics are constantly necessary.

It is well documented that mental health and related diagnoses damage credibility, and not enough is known about psychogenic symptoms and how their diagnosis correlates to erroneously held attitudes toward certain patients. Having a mental health diagnosis; being a women or other gender or sexual minority; and/or having a low socioeconomic status can mean lower quality of care across care settings—even when many or even most physicians have the best of intentions. As well, some health disparities are accounted for in material realities, such as proximity to premier care institutions, access to elite insurance policies, and abundance of disposable funds to pay for advanced care. While these demographics are changeable, altering material conditions is notoriously slow, difficult work. Dauntingly, too, the work toward more material justice is work that might not ever end, as forms of disenfranchisement seem to multiply over time, as global resources continue to shrink, and as wealth becomes more and more concentrated in the hands of an elite few. Discursive behaviors that lend themselves to credibility (or not) can be altered in real time and can help individuals in diverse circumstances get the best care possible. If we hope to empower the too-often voiceless, if we hope to learn "how better to hear our vernacular publics and encourage their participation in public life" (Troup, 2009, p. 452), we must find ways to cull their everyday rhetorical performances for potent theories worth proliferation. Chapters 3, 4, and 5 argue that there are an abundance of such performances worth analyzing.

Notes

1. While health disparities can refer to general differences in instances of disease and health outcomes in patient populations, health inequities refer explicitly to needless and preventable differences. For a discussion of this difference, see: www.bphc.org/whatwedo/health-equity-social-justice/what-is-health-equity/Pages/Health-Disparities-vs.-Health-Inequities.aspx.
2. These beliefs are often negatively impacted by racism, classism, sexism, and/ or gender discrimination.
3. It is worth noting that there is also robust data in interdisciplinary health literature to suggest that patients make biased assumptions about physicians for similar marks of difference (in race, class, gender, and social class).
4. Just as "there will be substantial social, economic and scientific costs if we cannot improve the diversity of our biomedical research workforce" (Economou, 2014, p. 1063), the consequences of lack of diversity in highly trained medical staff poses problems for patients, as having intersectional marks of difference yourself makes it perhaps less likely that you'd perpetuate myths based on race, class, or gender.
5. Chapter 3 will show that many of my interview participants also relied on a family member or partner to advocate for better care for them. I call this phenomenon "the credibility proxy."
6. This thread in and of itself is a rich source of empirical evidence of gender-based biases in clinical settings.
7. Importantly, this assumed lack of credibility is often attributable to reasons that exceed the discursive substance of the clinical dialogue, such as the person's age, race, class, education level, or income level.
8. Other examples of anti-stigma initiatives include: Time to Change (England); Opening Minds / Mental Health Commission of Canada; One of Us (Denmark); beyondblue (Australia); Sane (Australia); Like Minds Like Mine (New Zealand); California Mental Health Services Authority (USA); The Carter Center's Mental Health Program (USA); Association for the Improvement of Mental Health Programmes (Switzerland); Bring Change 2 Mind (USA); Time to Change Wales; See Change (Ireland); Northern Ireland Association for Mental Health; Hjärnkoll (Sweden); Obertament (Catalonia, Spain); 1decada4 (Andalusia, Spain); and Samen Sterk Zonder Stigma (the Netherlands).
9. As Chapter 3 will make clear, the DSM-V revisions to this diagnostic category included a stipulation that symptoms need not be unexplainable by physical/medical reasons, but that patients' level of impairment/distress be used to determine psychopathology. That said, the diagnosis is still used formally and informally when physical causes of distress cannot be found. The revision was meant to mitigate the possibility of ignoring signs of physical disease when symptoms are mysterious and/or evade obvious diagnosis.
10. Readers might wonder why Masterson did not consider that perhaps her high level of social capital born of having a doctoral degree would protect

her against the "worried well" label, but data in Chapter 3 will make it clear that her assessment of the possibility of being doubted despite some markers of credibility was accurate.

References

Adorjan, M., Christensen, T., Kelly, B., & Pawluch, D. (2012). Stockholm syndrome as vernacular resource. *The Sociological Quarterly, 53*(3), 454–474. doi:10.1111/j.1533-8525.2012.01241.x.

Alarcón, R. D. (2009). Culture, cultural factors and psychiatric diagnosis: Review and projections. *World Psychiatry: Official Journal of the World Psychiatric Association (WPA), 8*(3), 131–139. doi:10.1002/j.2051-5545.2009.tb00233.x.

APA. (2013). DSM-5 fact sheet: Somatic symptom disorder. Retrieved from www.psychiatry.org/psychiatrists/practice/dsm/educational-resources/dsm-5-fact-sheets

Bhargava, M. (2019). Perspective: What happens when the doctor blames you for your own cancer? Retrieved from www.washingtonpost.com/outlook/what-happens-when-the-doctor-blames-you-for-your-own-cancer/2019/01/11/2791611e-14ff-11e9-90a8-136fa44b80ba_story.html

Bowman, K., Telem, D. A., Hernandez-Rosa, J., Stein, N., Williams, R., & Divino, C. M. (2010). Impact of race and socioeconomic status on presentation and management of ventral hernias. *Archives of Surgery, 145*(8), 776–780. doi:10.1001/archsurg.2010.141.

Busby, L. P., Courtier, J. L., & Glastonbury, C. M. (2018). Bias in radiology: The how and why of misses and misinterpretations. *Radiographics: A Review Publication of the Radiological Society of North America, Inc, 38*(1), 236–247. doi:10.1148/rg.2018170107.

Chapman, E. N., Kaatz, A., & Carnes, M. (2013). Physicians and implicit bias: How doctors may unwittingly perpetuate health care disparities. *Journal of General Internal Medicine, 28*(11), 1504–1510. doi:10.1007/s11606-013-2441-1.

Clark, K. Why I believe racial bias in medicine almost killed my baby. Retrieved from https://themighty.com/2018/08/racial-bias-emergency-room/

Cockerham, W. C. (2016). *Sociology of mental disorder*. New York: Taylor & Francis.

Cuevas, A. G., O'Brien, K., & Saha, S. (2017). What is the key to culturally competent care: Reducing bias or cultural tailoring? *Psychology & Health, 32*(4), 493–507. doi:10.1080/08870446.2017.1284221.

Daugherty, S. L., Blair, I. V., Havranek, E. P., Furniss, A., Dickinson, L. M., Karimkhani, E., . . . Masoudi, F. A. (2017). Implicit gender bias and the use of cardiovascular tests among cardiologists. *Journal of the American Heart Association, 6*(12). doi:10.1161/JAHA.117.006872.

Dougall, J. L., & Schwartz, R. C. (2011). The influence of client socioeconomic status on psychotherapists' attributional biases and countertransference reactions. *American Journal of Psychotherapy, 65*(3), 249–265. doi:10.1176/appi.psychotherapy.2011.65.3.249.

Druckman, J. N., Trawalter, S., Montes, I., Fredendall, A., Kanter, N., & Rubenstein, A. P. (2018). Racial bias in sport medical staff's perceptions of others' pain. *The Journal of Social Psychology, 158*(6), 721–729. doi:10.1080/00224545.2017.1409188.

Dunham, L. (2018, February 14). In her own words: Lena Dunham on her decision to have a hysterectomy at 31. *Vogue.* Retrieved from www.vogue.com/article/lena-dunham-hysterectomy-vogue-march-2018-issue

Economou, J. S. (2014). Gender bias in biomedical research. *Surgery, 156*(5), 1061–1065. doi:10.1016/j.surg.2014.07.005.

Fassler, J. (2015). How doctors take women's pain less seriously. Retrieved from www.theatlantic.com/health/archive/2015/10/emergency-room-wait-times-sexism/410515/

Haider, A. H., Schneider, E. B., Sriram, N., Dossick, D. S., Scott, V. K., Swoboda, S. M., . . . Freischlag, J. A. (2015). Unconscious race and social class bias among acute care surgical clinicians and clinical treatment decisions. *JAMA Surgery, 150*(5), 457–464. doi:10.1001/jamasurg.2014.4038.

Haider, A. H., Schneider, E. B., Sriram, N., Scott, V. K., Swoboda, S. M., Zogg, C. K., . . . Cooper, L. A. (2015). Unconscious race and class biases among registered nurses: Vignette-based study using implicit association testing. *Journal of the American College of Surgeons, 220*(6), 1086.e3. doi:10.1016/j.jamcollsurg.2015.01.065.

Haider, A. H., Sexton, J., Sriram, N., Cooper, L. A., Efron, D. T., Swoboda, S., . . . Cornwell, E. E. (2011). Association of unconscious race and social class bias with vignette-based clinical assessments by medical students. *Jama, 306*(9), 942–951. doi:10.1001/jama.2011.1248.

Henningsen, P. (2016). *Fear of flying: Relying on the absence of organic disease in functional somatic symptoms.* http://doi.org/10.1016/j.jpsychores.2016.07.007.

Hinshaw, S. P. (2006). *The mark of shame: Stigma of mental illness and an agenda for change.* New York: Oxford University Press.

Hirsh, A. T., Hollingshead, N. A., Ashburn-Nardo, L., & Kroenke, K. (2015). The interaction of patient race, provider bias, and clinical ambiguity on pain management decisions. *The Journal of Pain: Official Journal of the American Pain Society, 16*(6), 558–568. doi:10.1016/j.jpain.2015.03.003.

Hoffmann, D. E., & Tarzian, A. J. (2001). The girl who cried pain: A bias against women in the treatment of pain. *Journal of Law, Medicine, and Ethics, 29*, 13–27. doi:10.2139/ssrn.383803. Retrieved from https://papers.ssrn.com/abstract=383803

Hoffman, K. M., Trawalter, S., Axt, J. R., & Oliver, M. N. (2016). Racial bias in pain assessment and treatment recommendations, and false beliefs about biological differences between blacks and whites. *Proceedings of the National Academy of Sciences of the United States of America, 113*(16), 4296–4301. doi:10.1073/pnas.1516047113.

Hymel, K. P., Laskey, A. L., Crowell, K. R., Wang, M., Armijo-Garcia, V., Frazier, T. N., . . . Weeks, K. (2018). Racial and ethnic disparities and bias in the evaluation and reporting of abusive head trauma. *The Journal of Pediatrics, 198*, 143. e1. doi:10.1016/j.jpeds.2018.01.048.

Jenell Johnson. (2010). *The skeleton on the couch: The Eagleton affair, rhetorical disability, and the stigma of mental illness.* Routledge. doi:10.1080/02773945.2010.517234.

Jutel, A. (2010). Medically unexplained symptoms and the disease label. *Social Theory & Health, 8*(3), 229–245. doi:10.1057/sth.2009.21.

Kalin, J., & Gruber, D. (2018). Gut rhetorics: Toward experiments in living with microbiota. *Rhetoric of Health & Medicine, 1*(3–4), 269–295. doi:10.5744/rhm.2018.1014.

Katz, J., Rosenbloom, B. N., & Fashler, S. (2015). *Chronic pain, psychopathology, and DSM-5 somatic symptom disorder.* Los Angeles, CA: SAGE Publications. doi:10.1177/070674371506000402.

Kentner, A. C., & Grace, S. L. (2017). Between mind and heart: Sex-based cognitive bias in cardiovascular disease treatment. *Frontiers in Neuroendocrinology, 45,* 18–24. doi:10.1016/j.yfrne.2017.02.002.

Keränen, L. (2014). This weird, incurable disease: Competing diagnoses in the rhetorics of Morgellons. In T. Jones, D. Wear, & L. Friedman (Eds.), *Health humanities reader* (pp. 36–51). New Brunswick: Rutgers University Press.

Maina, I. W., Belton, T. D., Ginzberg, S., Singh, A., & Johnson, T. J. (2018). A decade of studying implicit racial/ethnic bias in healthcare providers using the implicit association test. *Social Science & Medicine, 199,* 219–229. doi:10.1016/j.socscimed.2017.05.009.

Masterson, S. (2018). *How I went from being seen as a 'worried well' to being diagnosed.* Retrieved from https://themighty.com/2018/07/worried-well-childhood-symptoms-diagnosed-as-adult/

Munch, S. (2004). Gender-biased diagnosing of women's medical complaints: Contributions of feminist thought, 1970–1995. *Women & Health, 40*(1), 101–121. doi:10.1300/J013v40n01_06.

Oliver, M. N., Wells, K. M., Joy-Gaba, J. A., Hawkins, C. B., & Nosek, B. A. (2014). Do physicians' implicit views of African Americans affect clinical decision making? *Journal of the American Board of Family Medicine: JABFM, 27*(2), 177–188. doi:10.3122/jabfm.2014.02.120314.

Pereda, B., & Montoya, M. (2018). Addressing implicit bias to improve cross-cultural care. *Clinical Obstetrics and Gynecology, 61*(1), 2–9. doi:10.1097/GRF.0000000000000341.

Pescosolido, B. A., Martin, J. K., Long, J. S., Medina, T. R., Phelan, J. C., & Link, B. G. (2010). "A disease like any other"? A decade of change in public reactions to schizophrenia, depression, and alcohol dependence. *The American Journal of Psychiatry, 167*(11), 1321–1330. doi:10.1176/appi.ajp.2010.09121743.

Pescosolido, B. A., Medina, T. R., Martin, J. K., & Long, J. (2013). The "backbone" of stigma: Identifying the global core of public prejudice associated with mental illness. *American Journal of Public Health, 103*(5), 853–860. doi:10.2105/AJPH.2012.301147.

Pettit, K. E., Turner, J. S., Kindrat, J. K., Blythe, G. J., Hasty, G. E., Perkins, A. J., . . . Cooper, D. D. (2017). Effect of socioeconomic status bias on medical student-patient interactions using an emergency medicine simulation. *AEM Education and Training, 1*(2), 126–131. doi:10.1002/aet2.10022.

Prendergast, C. (2001). On the rhetoric of mental disability. In J. C. Wilson (Ed.), *Embodied rhetoric: Disability in language and culture* (pp. 47–60). Carbondale: Southern Illinois University Press.

Rowe, C. (2018). Living with schizoaffective disorder in the world of academia. Retrieved from https://themighty.com/2018/04/going-to-college-grad-school-with-schizoaffective-disorder/

Samulowitz, A., Gremyr, I., Eriksson, E., & Hensing, G. (2018). "Brave men" and "emotional women": A theory-guided literature review on gender bias in health care and gendered norms towards patients with chronic pain. *Pain Research & Management, 2018,* 6358624. doi:10.1155/2018/6358624.

Saposnik, G., Redelmeier, D., Ruff, C. C., & Tobler, P. N. (2016). Cognitive biases associated with medical decisions: A systematic review. *BMC Medical Informatics and Decision Making, 16*(1), 138. doi:10.1186/s12911-016-0377-1.

Schumann, J. H. (2017). After Charlottesville, A doctor reflects on hateful patients and his own biases. Retrieved from www.npr.org/sections/health-shots/2017/08/16/543883816/after-charlottesville-a-doctor-reflects-on-hateful-patients-and-his-own-biases

Schwartz, R. C., & Blankenship, D. M. (2014). Racial disparities in psychotic disorder diagnosis: A review of empirical literature. *World Journal of Psychiatry, 4*(4), 133. doi:10.5498/wjp.v4.i4.133.

Smedley, B. D., Stith, A. Y., & Nelson, A. R. (2003). *Unequal treatment: Report of the institute of medicine on racial and ethnic disparities in healthcare.* Washington, DC: The National Academies Press.

Spector, N. (2017). Lady gaga has fibromyalgia. what is it? Retrieved from www.nbcnews.com/better/health/lady-gaga-has-fibromyalgia-what-it-ncna803046

St. Amant, K. S. (2017). The cultural context of care in international communication design: A heuristic for addressing usability in international health and medical communication. *Communication Design Quarterly Review, 5*(2), 62–70. doi:10.1145/3131201.3131207.

Susan's Story: See me is Scotland's programme to tackle mental health stigma and discrimination. Retrieved from www.seemescotland.org/stigma-discrimination/personal-stories/personal-stories/susans-story/

Teachman, B. A., & Brownell, K. D. (2001). Implicit anti-fat bias among health professionals: Is anyone immune? *International Journal of Obesity, 25*(10), 1525–1531. doi:10.1038/sj.ijo.0801745.

The Mighty: We face disabilities and diseases together. Retrieved from https://themighty.com

Troup, C. L. (2009). Ordinary people can reason. *Journal of Business Ethics, 87*(4), 441–453.

Tsai, J., Brooks, K., DeAndrade, S., Ucik, L., Bartlett, S., Osobamiro, O., . . . George, P. (2018). Addressing racial bias in wards. *Advances in Medical Education and Practice, 9*, 691–696. doi:10.2147/AMEP.S159076.

Vincent, L. (2017). Me, lady gaga, and the medical establishment that failed us both. Retrieved from www.thecut.com/2017/09/me-lady-gaga-and-the-doctors-that-failed-us-both.html

Weiss, S. (2018, October 16). Women with chronic illnesses: How long & how many doctors did it take you to get diagnosed?. Retrieved from https://twitter.com/suzannahweiss/status/1052249111225720832?lang=en

Williams, R. L., Romney, C., Kano, M., Wright, R., Skipper, B., Getrich, C. M., . . . Zyzanski, S. J. (2015). Racial, gender, and socioeconomic status bias in senior medical student clinical decision-making: A national survey. *Journal of General Internal Medicine, 30*(6), 758–767. doi:10.1007/s11606-014-3168-3.

3   Contested Diagnoses and *Ethos*
How Patients Push Back When Care Providers Misdiagnose Somatic Symptoms

Introduction

Gretchen,[1] a young international affairs professional living in Scotland and a participant in the interview research[2] that is explored in this chapter, sought out medical care when she began to experience a range of "very worrying symptoms," including "severe pain all over [her] body, neurological symptoms such as muscle twitching, vision changes, and digestive distress"—symptoms that came on "overnight." As she explained, "My heart rate and my blood pressure would spike up . . . I was hospitalized for the first two weeks and nobody could figure out what was going on."

Despite her insistence that something physical was causing her symptoms, care providers in the hospital where she'd been admitted due to the severity of her state insisted that these things were "all in her head"—a devastating reality. As she recalled:

> I didn't know how to convince them that I wasn't "crazy," you know, that I didn't have some history of covered up psychological issues or that I wasn't having a psychotic break and that's terrifying that you cannot convince people. There's no possible way in the world to convince people that you're sane. It doesn't make sense.

Two years[3] and 20 doctors later, Gretchen finally knew her symptoms were actually the result of two related conditions: autoimmune small fiber neuropathy and autonomic neuropathy. Speaking on the long road to diagnosis and the difficulty of overcoming the initial assessment of her symptoms as "in her head," she commented, "Once the first round of tests come back negative, or not showing what it was they thought it was, then they would start doubting my experience, my reputation." Her assessment of her situation is an astute one; she indicated that reaching a place where she could get appropriate care meant overcoming care providers' anchoring bias (care providers' unwillingness to abandon initial diagnoses despite evidence that another explanation is likely or at least plausible) in favor of a psychological explanation for her symptoms and that having symptoms for which there are no easy answers leads to a sharp and swift loss of credibility. My conversation with her and with 67 others convinces me that those who do manage to successfully navigate care settings when symptoms evade easy answers rely on strong appeals to *ethos* in their journeys to appropriate care. In fact, I coded[4] 180 references to being misdiagnosed in 60 of the 68 interviews and coded 51 references to biases and judgments due to demographic markers in 24 interviews.

With medical mistrust linked to poor communication with providers and to low levels of health literacy (White et al., 2016), many have argued that "appropriate, effective, and nuanced communication between patients and physicians is the bedrock on which all healthcare is based" (Kornelsen, Atkins, Brownell, & Woollard, 2016, p. 375). Much of this literature focuses on the need to educate healthcare providers on best practices for effectively communicating with their patients. The need for strong, working "relationships between providers and patients is well documented in both the medical and sociology literature, as well as in the discourse of rhetoricians and communication researchers" (Young & Flower, 2002, p. 75). For some researchers, improving patient-provider communication and collaboration is a means to increasing compliance (see, for example, Schwartz et al., 2017). Less attention has been given to strategies patients might use to successfully communicate with their care providers, and these strategies, I argue, are discernable in patients' everyday exchanges with their care teams.

In their film *Unrest*, Dryden and Brea (2017) document Brea's long and arduous journey to diagnosis with and seeking out effective treatment for chronic fatigue syndrome. Important texts like this film show that for the long-term misdiagnosed and undiagnosed, clinical conversations become increasingly routine parts of everyday life. Time can seem to fold in on itself. Hours and days become weeks, months, and years of wading through disruptive symptoms despairing for answers—all while trying to keep employment and personal life as intact as possible. Desperation and hopelessness are especially difficult to avoid when no one seems to take the symptoms seriously.

Mapping the appeals to *ethos* that might undermine anchoring and other biases in clinical settings is important since, unfortunately, experiences like Gretchen's are far from unique. In some cases, the consequences of misdiagnosis of psychogenic symptoms are long-term damage to organs or body systems due to lack of treatment for a medical illness. In extreme cases, though, these are quite literally matters of life and death. For example, when 37-year-old UK professor Lisa Smirl[5] went to several physicians to seek out treatment for a range of unusual symptoms, she was told that they were "all in her head" and the result of anxiety and depression. Smirl was, thus, put on antidepressants and experienced no relief. In fact, over the course of a year, her symptoms worsened until, finally, a physician sent her for the chest x-ray that would reveal Smirl's true affliction: metastatic lung cancer (Duff, 2012, n.p.).

The gap in time between her initial visits to clinics for help and the actual diagnosis, unfortunately, meant that her case was terminal. Remarkably, though, Smirl was relieved and vindicated when she got her diagnosis and was sure that her status as a middle-aged woman interfered with doctors' ability to take her symptoms seriously.

Particularly for those initially misdiagnosed with symptoms "in their heads," a diagnosis of a physical condition means vindication and a restoration of the credibility that had been called into question when their subjective symptoms reports were disparaged. As these cases and the data I report on in this chapter also show, accurate diagnosis can rely heavily on a person's ability to overcome care providers' initial assessment of psychogenic symptoms. Once that work is done, many patients are moved to share their experiences.

Smirl was moved to write about her experiences so that others could learn from her *mis*diagnosis. In a blog post, she expressed her frustration at doctors' unwillingness to consider her symptoms as signs of physical disease and implored readers:

> It is so easy to say that someone's symptoms are "anxiety" related if they are a little bit complicated, unclear or unusual. Don't repeat my mistakes. You know when something is wrong. Find another doctor that you connect with and who takes your concerns seriously. Get referrals. Get tested. Refuse to be dismissed.
>
> (Duff, 2012, n.p.)

In response to this call to action, another woman commented: "I was point blank asked by a neurologist that I was seeing for some unusual symptoms of lung cancer … whether or not I might be a hypochondriac" (Duff, 2012, n.p.). Stories like Smirl's, which are dauntingly common (Kennedy, 2012), highlight the stigmatizing nature of psychogenic[6] diagnoses as well as the relationship between assumed lack of credibility and inadequate care.

Popular press coverage of this important issue points out significant gender bias in medical research and training—issues that also contribute to this problem (Dusenbery, 2018b; Levy, 2018). While Smirl used blog posts to share her experiences, others have used social media to call attention to this issue. As Yahoo Style UK writer Fowler (2018) explained:

> There are sure to be plenty of women who would raise their hand if asked whether their doctor has ever dismissed their health concerns. For too long, a large majority of us have put off booking an appointment for period pain or anxiety through fear of being laughed out

of the door. Now, women are taking back the control through the power of social media.

(n.p.)

As mentioned in the previous chapter, Journalist Weiss (2018) posted about her experiences with misdiagnosis of a chronic illness on Twitter with the message:

Women with chronic illnesses: how long & how many doctors did it take you to get diagnosed? I counted 11 months & 17 doctors & wrote down what each did to show what we go through just to begin to heal.

(n.p.)

Weiss's post was popular, if not quite viral; it elicited 429 retweets, 390 comments, and 975 likes. Commenters, of course, told similar stories of having symptoms dismissed as "in their heads" prior to obtaining an accurate medical diagnosis.

Despite the encouraging nature of such activist work, as Dubriwny (2013) explained, "disrupting hegemonic media messages about women's health" is "no easy task" (p. 188), and one such message is that women's pain is not to be trusted and that women are more likely than men to suffer from psychogenic symptoms. These cases, thus, underscore the fact that accurate diagnosis carries significant symbolic meaning—even in cases where there is no hope for a cure or an effective treatment. The diagnostically unmoored move from appointment to appointment, from diagnostic test to diagnostic test, all while trying to maintain life as usual alongside the emotional fallout from having those symptoms doubted and dismissed.[7] Establishing and maintaining strong *ethos* in such circumstances, of course, is no easy task. As their *ethos*-building strategies will show, the interview participants I was fortunate enough to speak with overcame the self-doubt that inevitably accompanied their misdiagnosis. Moreover, when care providers they trusted suggested that their symptoms had no physical causes, many diligently pursued mental health interventions expecting to see symptoms improvement. The fact that mental health-related care plans did not lessen symptoms helped to reassure them that something physical was going on, but these processes took months to years to decades.

Chapters 1 and 2 make it clear that chronic mental illnesses are notoriously stigmatizing and often lead to social isolation, homelessness, and unemployment (Johnson, 2010), so it is unsurprising that the assumption of mental health issues in the medically ill makes it more difficult for them to be taken seriously and to get adequate treatment for physical problems. Moreover, Chapter 2 especially shows that gender, race, and class-based biases are frequent in clinical settings where symptoms labelled "in the patient's head" can mask treatable diseases. In fact, disenfranchised populations are more likely than those with social capital to be misdiagnosed and, thus, to continue to suffer or even die from treatable medical problems (Castro, Carbonell, & Anestis, 2012; Chapman, Kaatz, & Carnes, 2013; Hoffman & Tarzian, 2001; Graham, 2015; Ladwig, Marten-Mittag, Erazo, & Gündel, 2001; Novella, 2009; Wool & Barsky, 1994). Undoubtedly, what a care provider believes to be true of a patient's credibility impacts the kind of care they will get. While implicit biases (as discussed in Chapter 2, instances where a care provider might exhibit race-, class-, or gender-based biases without having conscious awareness of those biases) stack the deck against certain patients at the outset, participants in the study reported on in this chapter have developed savvy rhetorical tactics to bolster their credibility in everyday clinical encounters such that their medical conditions were eventually acknowledged.[8]

What is also likely clear from the first two chapters is that this book is about rhetorical *ethos* and its capacity to illuminate and potentially posit interventions for the biases that operate on the level of and just below discourse; that erupt in embodied, day-to-day interactions; and that call attention to the problematic binary between bodies and minds that pervade contemporary biomedical frameworks. Arguing that vernacular appeals to rhetorical *ethos* might interfere with the steady hum of stigma that casts its shadow over the lived experiences of bodies and minds, it theorizes *ephemeral rhetorical moves* as important sites of new meaning-making. In line with the scholarship on rhetorics of the vernacular and rhetorics of the everyday discussed in Chapter 1, I define "ephemeral rhetorical moves" as evanescent, on-the-spot rhetorical appeals that take energy and exigence from bodies and bodies of knowledge that are, as Teston (2017) pointed out, perpetually in flux—an admission that also leads to the insight that "knowledge is always contingent" (p. 8). Ephemeral rhetorical moves might emerge and disappear in rather unremarkable, everyday exchanges, but they are often recoverable via generative conversation. Once recovered, they accrete and suggest new theories.

In this chapter, these themes are explored through the accounts of women's and men's everyday experiences in clinical settings where they've sought out care for complicated symptoms and conditions to varying degrees of success. When they've managed to cultivate the savvy approaches to bolstering their *ethos*, they've, in many cases, gained accurate diagnoses of medical diseases. Diagnosis, of course, means entry into communities—vibrant, interested, engaged networks that care very much about finding successful treatments or even cures. These communities also take the need to provide support, guidance, and advocacy very seriously, and, thus, can be invaluable to those who've long been living with mysterious and debilitating symptoms. Indeed, advocacy communities can be vital resources for those who are struggling to persuade providers that their symptoms have been misdiagnosed and that they need additional care to discover the sources of their suffering.

Importantly, for many of the 68 people I was fortunate enough to speak with about their experiences seeking out care for difficult to diagnose conditions, their journeys have been long and arduous, and their creative appeals to *ethos* have helped them to navigate anchoring bias. In the case of most of my participants, of course, the "anchor" was a diagnosis of symptoms that were "in their heads," and their care providers were steadfast in their beliefs in those initial diagnoses. Ephemeral appeals to *ethos* also helped them to overcome implicit biases. Significantly, through these appeals to *ethos*, they've found community and have developed tactics for becoming their own (and, in some cases, others') advocates.

This discussion would be remiss without mentioning that the data shared in this chapter complicates body-mind dualism. Thus, part of the findings reported on in this chapter showcase everyday rhetorical tactics by which those suspected of mental health issues are vindicated when they are able to arrive—often through a lot of their own efforts—at accurate medical diagnoses. Many participants have no history of mental health issues; their symptoms were eventually wholly attributable to physical causes. That reality, though, does not mean that their medical care experiences have not led to significant psychological suffering. As well, others pointed out that what they see as their accurate, documented mental-health-issues profiles allowed care providers to ignore the presence of physical disease in favor of psychogenic diagnoses. Thus, even beyond exploring ways that individuals can overcome credibility issues that come with assumed psychogenic symptoms to arrive at accurate medical diagnoses, there is still room for more work on ending stigmas and abuses from which those with indelible marks of difference or disabilities, such as those with severe mental health differences or visible physical disabilities like limb loss, struggle daily. Such are the themes of Chapters 4 and 5.

Participant Recruitment, Methods, Limitations

The study I describe in this chapter used snowball sampling[9] and a survey[10] to recruit participants directly from online advocacy and activist spaces (official organization websites as well as social media sites) dedicated to medical conditions that are notoriously difficult to diagnose and/or commonly misdiagnosed as psychogenic, such as lupus and other autoimmune diseases, celiac disease, and endometriosis.[11] Working directly with these advocacy organizations made it possible to cast a wide net through which I was able to speak with a range of participants from various racial/ethnic backgrounds, a diversity of age groups, and from a variety of socioeconomic classes.[12] That said, participants were mostly women, as only three of the 68 interviewees were men. The gender imbalance has a few possible explanations. First, endometriosis is, of course, a disease that only affects women. Lupus is also more common in women and in women of color specifically. As well, Chapter 2 makes it clear that gender impacts the likelihood that a person will have had experiences being misdiagnosed with psychogenic symptoms. Thus, while the study would be more replete with more male participants, the imbalance is not a surprising outcome.

With the exception of two hearing impaired participants who'd requested emailed questions and the opportunity to respond in writing, interviews took place over the phone and were audio-recorded. Once transcribed, participants had the opportunity to amend any of their statements or to otherwise make corrections. Interview questions were designed to gather narrative accounts of participants' experiences with gaining accurate medical diagnoses when psychogenic symptoms were erroneously suspected. As a way to protect anonymity as much as possible, I did not ask interviewees to reveal their age, race/ethnicity, location, sexual orientation, or social class. That said, many revealed these demographic markers over the course of answering questions. Surprisingly, though, having high levels of social capital (education, income, occupation, wealth), did not change participants' self-reported experiences with misdiagnosis. Interview questions were crafted to elicit accounts that would mirror the "locally situated and experiential approach" found in critical-rhetorical ethnography as it is designed to gather an "insider perspective on the lived advocacy of individuals" as they "struggle to persuade in public for changes in policy, social life, or other issues that affect them" (Hess, 2011, p. 128). Interviews were conducted in an open, conversational style. Participants shared detailed accounts of clinical encounters through which I culled appeals to rhetorical *ethos*.

Figure 3.1 shows the 7 questions used in all interviews. Importantly, interview questions were designed to make it clear to participants that they did not have to reveal anything about their health histories that they did not wish to share. Moreover, all participants were asked the same questions in the same order with minimal follow-up questions—an important measure to ensure that participants would not feel pressure to reveal more about a health and medical experience than they would voluntarily give over the course of answering the questions. Participants were also encouraged to "pass" on any questions they did not wish to answer or to answer "yes" or "no" if they preferred not to elaborate on any questions in particular.

As Figure 3.1 shows, questions 1 and 2 ask about experiences with difficult to diagnose symptoms and with being misdiagnosed with psychogenic symptoms. Question 3 asks about research practices prior to seeking out care. Questions 4 and 6 ask for participants' assessments of their experiences in care settings with an emphasis on whether or not they feel valued and well cared for. Question 5 asks about tactics for gaining diagnostic tests[13] with particular attention to responses that indicated

Interview Questions

1. Do you suffer from symptoms for which doctors and other care providers cannot find causes?
    a. If so, can you tell me more about that, to the extent that you are comfortable sharing?
2. Have your symptoms ever been misdiagnosed as "in your head"? In other words, has a care provider ever suggested that your symptoms had no physical cause, but then a physical cause was later found?
3. When you go to a doctor or other care provider, do you research your symptoms first on your own?
    a. If so, what kind of research do you do?
4. When you explain symptoms and issues to doctors and care providers, do you believe they value and respect your assertions?
    a. Do they take you seriously?
    b. If so, why do you think they do?
    c. If not, why not?
5. Do you ever have to convince your doctors or care providers to perform diagnostic tests?
    a. If so, how do you try to convince them, and are you successful?
6. Overall, describe your level of satisfaction with the care you receive from your doctors and other care providers.
    a. Do you feel your concerns and symptoms are adequately addressed?
7. Is there anything else you're willing to share about how you establish your credibility in conversations with doctors and other care providers?

Figure 3.1 Interview Questions for Patient Credibility Study

that the assessment of psychogenic symptoms were hastily diagnosed and, thus, no tests were initially offered/given. This question also helped to establish the fact that diagnostic tests, once successfully obtained, led to accurate diagnoses of medical disease.

Finally, question 7 served as a form of respondent validation. It asked participants to describe their tactics for establishing their credibility in conversations with doctors and other care providers in their own words as a way to honor vernacular commitments to participatory critical rhetoric as it "reconsiders the relationship between critic, rhetor, text/context, and audience" by "inviting new perspectives on these complex rhetorical processes" (Endres, Hess, Senda-Cook, & Middleton, 2016, p. 15).

That is, I wanted to hear my participants' own analyses of how they established their credibility after having symptoms doubted, to see how their responses mapped to my coding of their full interviews for appeals to *ethos*. The data I gathered via these interviews were ephemeral in two ways: 1) the interviewees recounted everyday encounters with a wide variety of care providers, often spanning many years (these conversations would otherwise be lost), and 2) the interviews themselves offered participants metacognitive space to articulate their rhetorical strategies in real time, in an extemporaneous fashion.

As I explain in Chapter 1, this chapter uses aspects of grounded theory, and, in so doing, honors the premise that "researchers can and should develop theory from rigorous analyses of empirical data. The analytic process consists of coding data; developing, checking, and integrating theoretical categories; and writing analytic narratives throughout inquiry" (Charmaz & Belgrave, 2015, p. 1). Likewise, it joins other studies that have used vernacular rhetoric as an analytic lens to examine gendered discourses (Bennett, 2014; Phillips, 2012). Taking the position that "effective rhetoric is evident even in the untrained vernacular of everyday social exchanges" (Ingraham, 2013, p. 9), considering that "the power to remake our everyday life resides, in part, in our capacities to see how rhetoric structures our lives and, in seeing, to craft anew our rhetorics" (Rai, 2016, p. 208), these interviews were analyzed to cull such successful rhetorical appeals.

While this data offered insight into what happens in a wide variety of clinical encounters, it is quite obviously not as illuminating as it would be to observe clinical conversations as an ethnographer. This limitation must be addressed, as despite the claim to capturing some ephemera, some important exchanges might be lost to memories of details, and firsthand providers' perspectives are absent. Still, I trust the veracity of these participants' statements and appreciate the density of data in particular with participants who've suffered through misdiagnosis with psychogenic symptoms. Much of the data below is shared from interviews with those who've reported that their symptoms were erroneously misattributed to psychological causes *before any other factors were explored*. Moreover, the appeals to *ethos* that emerged in this data have the benefit of hindsight and the depth of backstory that would not be readily available in observations made in clinical conversations. Still, the findings could productively be tested against ethnographic, clinical observations in the future. That is, future qualitative health researchers focused on patient-provider communication and miscommunication—particularly those interested in implicit bias and anchoring bias—might engage in observations of a series of clinical appointments. These observations could be examined via the lens of rhetorical *ethos*. Perhaps the coding scheme developed here would be usefully extended or even challenged with such data.

As noted in Chapter 1, the theoretical framework in the coding scheme below[14] generates middle-range theories. Explained Liehr and Smith (2017):

> Theories at the middle range level of discourse are described by the sociologist, Merton, as "those between the minor hypotheses of day to day research and unified theory." Thus, the middle range level is below the more philosophical or grand theories and above empirical generalizations framed as hypotheses.
>
> (p. 51)

An annotated example of how middle range theories are developed in health research can be found in Elo, Kääriäinen, Isola, & Kyngäs's (2013) study of wellness-supportive physical environments for housebound elderly. The authors use interview data to develop a theory that includes the insight that an "environment that enables safe activity" can lead to better health outcomes (p. 2). As they resist the finality of more established theories, middle-range theories can be used as the basis for further study; they are highly adaptable and exploratory. As such, they are especially appropriate for projects that seek to offer malleable preliminary inquiries into multifaceted problems.

Similarly, the appeals to *ethos* described here are related to *techne*—a term that refers to "creative skill," but also to "an art in the sense of a set of rules or theories" (Papillion, 1995, p. 149). As such, these appeals to *ethos* are exploratory and pliable and are very much meant to be adapted for other projects. As middle-range, they resist finality. In the sections below, I define each of these appeals to *ethos* and share especially strong examples from the data to support them.

To develop initial codes, I relied on two "first cycle" coding methods that are common in grounded theory: in vivo coding, or coding for actual words and phrases that reoccurred in the data (Saldaña, 2016, p. 105) and process coding, or examining the interviews for "routines and rituals of human life" (Saldaña, 2016, p. 111). While these methods, employed via NVivo software, yielded many viable codes, I needed to also implement second-cycle coding in the form of "pattern coding" to develop "explanatory or inferential codes" that could "identify an emerging theme, configuration, or explanation" (Saldaña, 2016, p. 236). This second cycle of coding helped me to develop an important insight: the data from this study indicates that when patients are successful in overcoming care providers' initial assessment of their symptoms as "in their heads," they do so via appeals to *ethos* that fit a three-part framework involving: 1) preparation, 2) performance, and 3) advocacy. In other words, they prepare for clinical appointments, they strategically perform in those appointments, and they advocate for themselves before, after, and between clinical encounters. Figure 3.2 shares the tactics—found in

Prepare for Clinical Appointments	Perform in Clinical Encounters	Become a Self-Advocate
Strategic Inquiry (textual research)	Assign a Credibility Proxy	Position Self as Own Advocate
Patient-to-Patient Networking (for research & support)	Emphasize day-to-day Impairment	Collaborate with Care Providers
Skilled Bodily Experimentation	Acknowledge Care Providers' Expertise & Use Strategic Hedging	Seek out a New Care Provider
Background Credibility Assessment	Perform Symptoms & Demonstrating Illness Severity	Make Proactive Health Decisions

Figure 3.2 Coding Scheme for Patient Credibility Study

first-cycle coding—through which they accomplish these three things. Importantly, as the data used to describe each of these approaches makes clear, they do not unfold in a linear way. Rather, those who've successfully overcome misdiagnoses of symptoms "in their heads" deploy these methods in recursive ways and often in tandem. Below, I define each aspect of the three-part coding scheme and offer examples of each to support their existence.

Prepare for Clinical Appointments

Participants made it clear that their journeys to appropriate medical-disease diagnoses came only after much preparation for the clinical appointments that would lead them to answers. Far from the clichéd and uncharitable notion of a "hysterical" cyberchondriac patient googling symptoms and arriving at a wildly inappropriate diagnosis, these interviewees engaged in high-quality textual research. In the process, they developed acute health and medical literacies (about research, etc.) and patients' strategies for presenting their health record file. Health literacy, once a term that referred almost exclusively to "people's ability to read and understand written information," is now used to name and describe "numerous factors that affect a person's ability to access, understand and use health information from many sources" (Batterham, Hawkins, Collins, Buchbinder, & Osborne, 2016, p. 3). In keeping with these logics, participants gathered vital information through

networking with other patients and engaged in what Kalin and Gruber (2018) have called, in relation to probiotics, "skilled experimentation," or "the impulse to create and engage in bodily experimentation"
(p. 286). That is, they used their knowledge of their body systems to try
out various food-based, medicinal, and movements-based protocols to
learn more about how their bodies might respond and to, thus, gather
important insight into what might be causing problematic symptoms.
These understandings included verifying that making moves to improve
mental well-being did not lessen symptoms, and thereby provided evidence that some physiological cause—some virus or clinically verifiable
disease—was present. Below, I feature examples of these tactics for preparing for clinical appointments to provide evidence of these maneuvers
as appeals to *ethos*.

Strategic Inquiry—High-Quality Textual Research

Emmons (2010) pointed out the dangers of discourses surrounding depression and their "multiple and changing definitions" as they lead to ambigu-
ities that engender "self-doctoring"[15] and lead many men and women to
critically examine their everyday behaviors for signs of pathology (p. 64).
In the same way, participants were aware of the misconception that they
and patients like them google random, unreliable health information and
reach hasty decisions on their health status on their own. Indeed, patients
with symptoms for which care providers cannot find obvious causes can
easily be labelled the "worried well"—overconsuming healthcare services
for imagined ailments and syndromes. Participants countered this misconception by displaying high levels of information literacy. Many interviewees rightly pointed out that they have learned not to expect the care
providers they go to for help to have advanced expertise in every possible
contingency or category of disease. Instead, they know that they need to
arm themselves with high-quality information prior to and after diagnoses
are made such that they can recover from the misconception that many
believe their care providers, at first, had of them: that they were aimlessly
and indiscriminately googling symptoms and latching on to improbable,
dire diagnoses. Of course, interviewees' backgrounds meant that they had
varying degrees of comfort with doing such research; while some reported
struggle, many more indicated that their educational backgrounds in
various areas helped them to make sense of dense information. I coded
145 items (ranging in length from a short phrase to a long paragraph)
in 62 interviews as "strategic inquiry—high-quality textual research."
Clearly, references to high-quality research were prevalent in this data.

Participants engaged in what one (Erin) called a "tremendous amount
of research," but they did not simply google their symptoms or consult

websites on the public web at random. Instead, they immersed themselves in "high-quality textual research" when they consulted, as they put it in typical interview responses: "The latest medical literature on PubMed" (Lucinda); "Information from the hospital library" (Leah); "Academic studies" (Selena); "Medical texts" (Beatrice); and "Medical journals" (Nia). This textual research in mostly peer-reviewed venues bolstered their credibility in clinical appointments when the existence of such research proved that they were not "hysterical" patients self-diagnosing based on weak evidence and inaccurate or outdated information on the public web.

Many participants researched symptoms to reach non-somatization diagnoses. However, they needed to perform effectively once in the clinical encounter to convince care providers that their self-assessments were accurate. Part of that process involved relaying the caliber of research in which they'd engaged. They also researched specific conditions once diagnosed, diagnostic tests and how to read lab results, care protocols to determine whether or not they'd adapt a pharmacological or surgical treatment, and diagnoses to learn more about alternative treatment options and lifestyle changes that could help.

Grace, for example, consulted "medical books" and in one, was able to find rare symptoms of celiac disease, which led to a long-awaited diagnosis of a physical cause for the skin rashes that had been misattributed to anxiety. As she put it, "I'm glad I stuck up for myself, but what if I didn't have that knowledge?"

While Grace's research helped her to identify a rare symptom of a well-known condition, Gretchen's research helped her to find classic symptoms of a rare autoimmune disease. As she explained, "I went straight to medical studies because it was sort of obvious to me that whatever I had wasn't necessarily common or easily identified because so many people and so many doctors had missed it, so I started looking through research and focusing really on medical research and recent releases of research." In the same way, another participant, Maris, finally was able to "get on to a diagnosis" of endometriosis by "self-diagnosing after doing [her] own research."

Although these participants' self-diagnoses were verified by doctors, others were more cautious about relying on textual research alone to self-diagnose. However, they still emphasized the value of high-quality research for aiding in credible clinical conversations. As the participant Laurine described, "I don't want to say, like, self-diagnose, but get as much information so I can ask really pointed questions and maybe point to things that, um, I wouldn't have thought of otherwise I guess, is the way I would put that."

Importantly, participants were often able to strategically bring up their research-based questions, ideas, and hunches in clinical conversations since the sources they relied on carried a credibility that they themselves were unfairly missing.

Notably, participants found that lost paper trails or convoluted digital records sometimes meant that a failure to read diagnostic test results led to misdiagnosis in the first place, so their own research into those results were tantamount to them finding a cause for symptoms. Some annotated existing patient health records, and others developed their own personal health records and files using symptoms and test results journals.[16]

Noting the importance of gaining literacy in diagnostic test results, the participant Isabella recommended to other patients: "Look up tests because you should." Others needed to research to get a diagnostic test approved in the first place, as with Dana, who does "extensive research" in "peer-reviewed science" and then prints off and highlights pertinent studies. She has had to bring this research with her to convince her doctor to recommend exploratory/diagnostic laparoscopy for what ended up being advanced (stage 4) endometriosis.

In describing how she prepares for clinical appointments, Julianne, another participant, similarly suggested that people treat doctor's appointments the way they'd treat a "job interview" or "an appointment for a bank loan, or, you know, going to buy a car" and advised that one must "do a little bit of homework about what's available" in terms of tests and treatments. Olivia's library-based research, too, focuses on "knowing the correct language" and "knowing about different tests." Others also research care protocols to determine whether or not they'd like to adapt a pharmacological or surgical treatment as well as to learn more about alternative treatment options and lifestyle changes that could help. Kathleen, for instance, makes use of PubMed for studies "on a procedure or a treatment or operation."

It is important to note that participants were quite clear that they see these research activities as attached to building and strengthening credibility in the clinical encounter. Lillian, for example, purposely brings information that is "credible to conventional doctors" to explain her health decisions. Just as Jeremy looks at "the latest studies," Glynis "arms [herself] with knowledge ahead of time" so that she can be "taken seriously." Sandra explained that she doesn't want to come across as "just some person who's just hysterical because all of this stuff they've read on the internet." As she explained in relation to her behaviors in the clinical encounter, "I'm more just like, 'This study, and that study, and this and that.' More sort of science and evidence-based stuff, not just anecdotal stuff." Commenting on the need to prepare for a clinical encounter, Ariana also explained that there are a lot of things "that aren't related to the appointment itself" that lead to being "credible," and a big part of that is "gathering data yourself."

This data shows that engaging in high-quality research empowers patients in clinical encounters—particularly when they are able to keep up-to-date on the latest findings related to their conditions. Annie explained that doctors "don't have the information [she does] on the disease." Katie similarly remarked, "I actually do have legitimate access to, like, real medical journals and studies and stuff, and, um, I would always try to keep that information in my head so then I'm there at the doctor and they are being dismissive I can say, 'Hey, you know I'm knowledgeable in this and you're not listening' type of thing." Stephanie, in the same way, emphasized the importance of gathering high-quality research ahead of clinical appointments: "I want to see. I want to see scientific proof, I want to say, 'Look, this is a definite thing and here's the proof,' so that I can take it with me and show the specialist. Otherwise, they won't listen to me."

If people with difficult-to-diagnose conditions can be misconstrued as the "worried well" or as merely anxious, then gaining advanced knowledge of symptoms, syndromes, and diagnostic tests via high-quality textual research and learning how best to present their findings to care providers helps them to bolster *ethos*, as the credibility of the sources they consult carries a credibility that they are missing. As well, they internalize discourse patterns that they then rely on when they go to a clinical appointment. Health literacy is embedded "in many health policies around the world," yet "it remains challenging to embed health literacy principles into routine practice" (Batterham et al., 2016, p. 3). These participants have found their own ways of doing this important work in their day-to-day lives.

Patient-to-Patient Networking for Research and Support

Recently, Executive Director of the National Network of Abortion Funds (NNAF) Yamani Yansá (2019) secured the top post in #blackwomentwitter with 27,430 likes and 10,051 retweets when she recounted how tweets with that hashtag helped her to learn to ask that refusals for diagnostic tests and treatments in clinical settings be documented in her chart—a move that often leads care providers to change their minds. Similarly, participants in the study explored in this chapter relied on social networks to learn tactics and gain knowledge through which they could acquire better care.

Dubriwny (2013) has argued that "effective women's health activism helps women form alternative ways of making sense of their lives" (p. 181), and the women and men[17] I interviewed indicated that they've garnered those benefits from the activist organizations they sought to network with post-diagnosis, those they found via seeking out answers to their symptoms, and those they became involved with after they successfully overcame care providers' beliefs that symptoms were "in their heads." Participants used their strong patient-to-patient networking to gather vital research as well as to find the kinds of support that empowered them to speak up for themselves in their clinical appointments. They gathered intel from those with the same symptoms or diagnoses. They also investigated treatment options others were using and looked into how others were faring on the medications they were prescribed and/or taking, and they used what they learned from their networks to counter care providers' suggestions that they consider outdated or even harmful treatment options. I coded 45 examples of networking for research and support in 24 interviews.

Gretchen used patient forums as a form of research into what might be causing her symptoms and found that her condition was an autoimmune one through a combination of that research and library-based research. As she put it, "I went through hours and hours and hours and hours of forums and different people talking about their different experiences and diseases and compared my own symptoms to theirs and causes and, you know, my lifestyle and different things." She focused on "entering support groups and seeing what patients [were] saying about their own experiences," such as "what tests worked for them, what medications worked for them, what the various names of conditions were, and what doctors they saw that were helpful." Though she cautioned that "there's a lot to wade through" and this form of inquiry yields information that is "not all helpful," she was clear that this research into others' experiences did, in her words, "eventually help me to get some of the language to be able to talk about these things, to look for different ways things were affecting me that I may not have noticed yet, and be able to write everything down and present it to my doctors in a way that made sense to them." Learning through these patient-to-patient networks, that is, she was able to improve her credibility in care settings and to effectively argue for the diagnostic tests that led to solving the origins of her mysterious symptoms.

In the same way, some participants share their educational backgrounds and attendant literacies by providing peer-reviewed research in patient-to-patient networks, as in Ella who reported, "So a lot of us do our own research and, and so we'll post scientific papers from peer-reviewed journals, and I find that really helpful. I have a science degree, I got a science degree before my law degree."

Physicians—even specialists in a particular area of medicine—cannot have time to accumulate the level of up-to-date, specific knowledge on a given condition, so networking to do good research becomes essential. Naturally, proving that you have more knowledge on a condition than the provider has the capacity to recover damaged *ethos*. Gaining this knowledge sometimes means consulting advocacy websites that synthesize bodies of research, as with Nina, who explained: "I use celiac sites that I am subscribed to that give me research updates, and that's usually where I'd go before I have a doctor's appointment related to this, because I trust their information."

Another important reason to research via patient networks is that physicians' understandings of precisely how a body will react to a medication or other treatment protocol is limited to the literature and to clinical observations, whereas patients themselves can comb through pages and pages of other patients' experiences in online forums and support groups such that their knowledge of what could happen to their bodies on a particular treatment plan is more replete. Indeed, Victoria commented that "You learn more with fellow people that have lupus." Selena "network[s] with some other people who have similar symptoms to find out what's worked for them," and Alyssa "talk[s] with other women that have the same symptoms and issues and get[s] educated on other treatments available and other people's experiences." Nia finds peer support and information from her "online group that's full of adults who have feeding tubes" and "that's been a resource for [her] because a lot of medical professionals don't know what it's like to actually have a tube and the ways that you can care for them at home." Amelia similarly commented, "I'm on several support groups on Facebook, and we're always on there asking, 'Have you ever had this happen?'" These participants can, thus, be ready to refute care providers' suggestions that the complications they experience are "in their heads." Sharing their familiarity with numerous other patients' firsthand accounts of bodily experiences, thus, bolsters their credibility.

Preparing for a clinical encounter via networking can also mean becoming empowered to refuse care providers' suggested treatment protocols and erroneous assumptions about the severity of disease or symptoms, which can be immensely important. Nikki explained this well:

> After the surgery, when the surgeon told me that I have endometriosis, he did tell me that birth control was an option and he kind of made it seem, "Oh, like, we could get it under control," but then I read stuff on an endometriosis Facebook group that that doesn't, that's not a way to go.

Rosa also commented: "I was an educated patient and knew that, basically, what she was telling me was not in any way, shape, or form helpful." When Dana "finally found a support group"—what she called "a very educational support group," she "learned way more" about the kinds of treatments she would accept than she had from interactions with providers.

Many also spoke to the importance of these networks as support spaces, as sources of strength and confidence—attributes that helped to create more powerfully compelling personas in office visits. In this way, these networks are similar to what bell hooks (1990) has referred to as "homeplaces" or "sites of resistance" that elevate spirits, reduce despair, and offer strength for struggles ahead (p. 385). As Maggie put it, "I found leaders in the industry, that ran blogs, and started following their blogs, and I found groups online, for support, and I find that support groups online are very helpful, from be it not necessarily a knowledge stand-point, but from a togetherness standpoint."

Speaking to the things she's learned, Kathleen explained:

> I do a lot of advocacy work, and I'm in good groups in support groups online and everything. Because people tend to minimize women's pain, and even in the ER, women wait 26 minutes longer on average than men to be seen. And women are often given Ativan or Halcion when they get to the ER when they're in pain because people just think they're hysterical.

These participants, thus, use the knowledge and support they gain in net-worked spaces to empower themselves to demand better care once they arrive at (or return to) what might be read as a hostile clinical setting—a place where they aren't always believed.

Skilled Bodily Experimentations

Another form of preparation for clinical encounters participants engaged in when their credibility had been compromised by the suggestion that their symptoms were "all in their heads" was by combining research with personal experimentation, which could even be more effective than research on its own for establishing *ethos*. These experiments range from intentional and based on research to wholly accidental. However, in all cases, participants used the results of their skilled bodily experimentation to offer empirical proof to their care providers that their physical symp-toms have physical—and not mental—causes. I coded 32 items "skilled bodily experimentation" in 18 interviews.

Not all skilled bodily experimentation is purposeful in terms of seek-ing out answers to perplexing symptoms, though it still provides useful information that helps to bolster credibility. An example of an accidental, though skilled, form of bodily experimentation can be found in Carina's interview. After eight years of unexplained skin rashes, many diagnoses of depression and anxiety as the underlying cause, and begging unsuc-cessfully for diagnostic tests (which, as a nurse, she knew quite a lot about), she stumbled upon evidence of the symptom's true cause. As she explained:

> Um, I actually had been on uh, like for weight loss, like a Paleo diet, um, for a few months at the beginning of this past, at the beginning of this past year. I told my doctor that I'd seen improvement in my skin symptoms, but then had been off that diet for, like, the last four months. And, and I think that's when I think the symptoms came back worse, and I think that's what made him decide to go ahead and test it because obviously I had been off of gluten for four months at

the beginning of the year and had lost 25 pounds. My symptoms had improved, and going back on it [gluten], my symptoms were back as bad, if not worse than ever. And I had done that research, and I told him I suspected I had a gluten allergy, and he said, "We'll, let's just test and see."

Predictably, then, Carina's experimentation with food led her to provide evidence to counter the care provider's assertion that her symptoms were "all in her head." Her credibility shifted because she could offer proof that a physical change led to significant symptoms improvement.

In the same way, Jamie arrived at the conclusion that her symptoms were related to her hormonal cycle rather than to psychosis; as she noted, "After I stopped breastfeeding, my symptoms got a lot worse."

Sharing results of skilled experimentation goes a long way in establishing the self as a diligent patient ready to do anything to find answers— even when none are available yet.

Not surprisingly, since the use of complementary and alternative medicines (CAM) took off in the 1990s, as explained in Derkatch (2016), participants have learned a lot about their own bodies via, as Selena put it, "exercise" and "changing [their] own diet," which Selena explained as "taking matters into [her] own hands." Using skilled experimentation, through "trial and error," she was able to determine that she is "extremely lactose intolerant." Others found ways to experiment with medications to find relief, such as Lillian, who mentioned: "I'm taking a medication that's off-label and see how it's working better as compared to what they suggest."

In an interesting case, Nora noted that her primary care doctor helped her to engage in skilled experimentation to convince the rheumatologist that her symptoms were not due to psychogenic causes, but were likely autoimmune:

He looked at me and he goes, "I don't normally do this," he said, "but I'm gonna give you a prescription for prednisolone. If it helps, you'll feel better within two weeks. If it does that, you probably have something called polymyalgia rheumatica, and you should go back to a rheumatologist and get followed up with it." And that's exactly what happened with that.

The fact that care providers find skilled bodily experimentations convincing and a patient's willingness to engage in them a sign of credibility, though, is likely linked to another finding of this interview research—that doctors, at times, suggest patients engage in self-care or experimental or holistic options when they believe the symptoms are in the patient's head. This can be a real source of frustration and can, in fact, lead participants to question their own skills in self-care.

Participants have heard, as Erin has, "[t]hings like, 'Well, if you won't even try acupuncture,' I'm like, 'Oh my gosh! I have a stack of records showing all the things that I've tried to do.'" Still, when a skilled bodily experimentation—intentionally related to the symptoms at hand or not—leads to evidence to back up a patients' claims, that increases their credibility, as does the mere mention of the things they are trying.

Background Credibility Assessment

My participants included several lawyers and healthcare workers, international affairs professionals, and a wide variety of academic and clinical scientists and social scientists. Yet, most reported that their background credibility—effective as a way to bolster *ethos* in other settings—was no help once their symptoms were attributed to psychological causes. I coded 57 examples of participants discussing the futility of using background credibility in clinical settings in 28 interviews.

As Timothy recalled of his mysterious symptoms and the journey to getting an accurate diagnosis of celiac disease, referencing his background in biochemistry didn't make any difference. Remarkably, then, appeals to careers or other background markers of professional or personal successes—even in the health sciences—are not always successful appeals to *ethos* once symptoms have been deemed "in your head" or, in his case, simply attributed to an "unknown topical allergy."

Many very powerful and accomplished women and men participated in this study. They've been especially engaged and proactive in their health and are trying to contribute to research that might improve health outcomes for women and other underserved persons.

As Gretchen explained:

> I am an academic [slight laugh], which I am very . . . which I am sure you understand, I am hyperrational. I try and be very objective when I look at things and try not to let my own fear about my health or, you know, what I am experiencing sway my understanding about things. And so I . . . so I would start telling doctors that, um, but then I realized that once you are in the patient role, that it doesn't matter kinda who you are outside of the office, outside of the doctor's office or outside of the hospital. And so, when nobody takes you seriously as a human, who's complaining of pain and issues, you move on to "you're a professional" and if nobody takes you seriously as a professional, your education, all of these things that are supposed to solidify your ability to represent yourself, when all of those things are gone, you're really at a loss as to how to get anyone to believe you or take you seriously.

Gretchen's sentiment captures many other utterances related to how background credibility was not usually helpful in clinical conversations once symptoms were believed to be "in your head." Taking stock and recognizing that background credibility was not helpful led many to turn to clinical performance to gain stronger *ethos*.

One of a few exceptions was Ella, who mentioned: "I often try to sneak into the conversation that I'm a lawyer, not just because I'm a lawyer, but because I have a lot of education, and I find they tend to take me more seriously, and think that, my sense is they think I'm less likely to be exaggerating or, um, just looking for attention."

Thus, participants assess their background credibility and its usefulness (or lack thereof) in bolstering *ethos* when symptoms are doubted. If background credibility is not helpful, strategic performances to gain stronger *ethos* become necessary.

Perform in Clinical Encounters

As the "prepare" coding examples and analyses make clear, preparation can lead to or be prompted by clinical performance; the arrangement is recursive rather than linear. These tactics accrete and overlap. They interweave in infinite combinations with no discernable patterns in terms of common pairings. However, what is clear in the data is that no participant was able to rely on a singular tactic; all used some combination. In this section, I share ways participants performed strong *ethos* in their clinical appointments. Some marks of performance were on a semiotic level, such as those who've tried to appear professional, well dressed, and/or older. Other performances rely more on linguistic-rhetorical skill to sway the clinical conversation in a direction where the patient is getting the care they need.

Patient-provider communication, of course, constitutes a vast area of interdisciplinary research in its own right. Studies posit effective, communicative interventions and methods for current healthcare workers and those in training such that better health outcomes are possible and patients and their caregivers are more satisfied with the care given. Other areas of emphasis include, for example, improving the efficiency of the clinical interview, etc. As Hernández and Dean (2019) explained, "The patient-provider interaction has generated significant scholarship over the last five decades, focusing on how medically authoritative power and clashes between experiential and biomedical knowledge shape patient-provider encounters" (n.p.). Indeed, the women in this interview study, as noted above, where well aware of these daunting realities. Some performative rhetorics to which they resorted were not all that empowering, yet they naturally emphasized the need to get better care at all cost.

The data I coded as related to clinical performance specifically highlights patients' strategies for establishing (or, in many cases, re-establishing) *ethos* once a care provider has deemed their subjective reports of what is happening with their bodies suspect, often due to the constructs

Hernández and Dean (2019) cited above. They do so by assigning what I am calling a "credibility proxy," or a person whose credibility has not been compromised, who's willing to vouch for the patient; by emphasizing day-to-day impairment to build empathy and understanding; by acknowledging care providers' expertise and making use of verbal hedging; and by performing and/or demonstrating the severity of symptoms via empirical proofs.

Assigning a Credibility Proxy

The power of reputation and the marks of credibility that precede/exceed the oratorical scene are long-standing features of rhetorical *ethos*, and what I am calling the "credibility proxy" is a tactic for gaining stronger *ethos* when credibility is doubted, via having a person with established *ethos* quite simply vouch for you as a credible source of clinically significant symptoms reports of conditions that have physical etiologies. Dusenbery's (2018a) work of feminist journalism found that women with a variety of health conditions "attested to the power of a male relative— whether a partner, a father, or even a son—to help ensure their symptoms were taken seriously" (p. 295). Participants in my study similarly described a range of proxies to enhance their credibility in clinical settings.

Layla, for example, explained this tactic simply in relation to gaining credibility via a proxy when symptoms are doubted: "Sometimes I take somebody with me who has seen the thing happen and they can prove it, too." In total, I coded 64 instances of the credibility proxy in 30 interviews.

While most credibility proxies that came up in interviews were loved ones (parents or intimate partners) that actually brought their credibility into the physical appointment, or ancillary healthcare workers on the scene to vouch for the patient, others, such as a new provider or a specialist who joins a care team, might use patient records, referrals, and test results to lend credence to patients' claims to physical ailments. That is, in some cases, technical documents stand in for the credibility proxy, creating a layering effect and a complexity of ontologies. In other cases, participants relied on family history—bodies elsewhere in space and time—to fill in for the speaker in real time, substantiating their concerns and witnessing to their suffering.

Nina, like others, relied on her mother as credibility proxy when her pituitary tumor was misdiagnosed as stress and anxiety: "My mother was the main um, convincer in that situation. She, we recently just sat down with my doctor and said, 'Look, she's still having this. We don't really care if you think it's stress. It has, it has a name and we're gonna figure out what it is.'"

Ella also relied on a parent as credibility proxy, noting:

> So, the last time I was in emergency with an endometriosis flare, she kind of pulled the doctor away and said, "You know, my daughter

has a really high pain tolerance. She's broken jaw bones, she had gallstones, she, you know, has a really high tolerance for pain," and that really, I think, that hit home for him, so I found having somebody else there to vouch for my pain tolerance level has helped some.

Katie found, unfortunately, that simply having a male present, even if he doesn't speak, helped her *ethos* by proxy. As she put it:

I take my husband with me who has no idea. Like he [the doctor] has to speak to him with medical stuff in the simplest way and in the simplest terms, but just being there at an appointment when I had an endometriosis appointment—just him being in the room even not saying anything—it felt like I was being listened to more, just having him there.

Similarly, Maggie recalled her experience bringing her husband as a credibility proxy: "I brought him as my character witness: 'I attest that my wife is not having panic attacks,' because I just felt like I wasn't being believed, and that's difficult."

While these interviewees relied on loved ones to enhance *ethos* by proxy, some participants relied on other care providers to serve as credibility proxies, as did Rita who explained, "I had a nurse practitioner at the free clinic or low-income clinic um, who knew something was wrong. She wasn't sure what it was, but she knew something was wrong. Ultimately, it was her persistence that got me the surgeon that finally took it seriously."

Shen, Hamann, Thomas, and Ostroff (2016) found that strong patient-provider communication correlated to lower levels of lung cancer stigma, and this finding is related to the potential of care providers as powerful credibility proxies. Kathleen, whose experience was quite similar to Rita's, put it simply: "Long story short, I found somebody who saved me, and now he makes other doctors listen." Of course, such arrangements are potentially tricky for the care providers involved, as they risk conflict with their colleagues. Perhaps that is why this form of *ethos* by proxy is often carried out via paperwork as opposed to in real-time debates.

Gretchen, though, noticed that a credibility proxy can be semi-present via clinical documents and the boost to *ethos* is just as effective: "Once I would bring the positive test results and the official diagnosis from another doctor back, they were much more inclined to help, to believe it, to listen."

That said, some care providers are willing to engage in conflict due to their convictions on best care. Sandra's longtime psychiatrist, for instance, has served as her credibility proxy when other care providers misattribute physical symptoms to her mental health. She explained:

My hair started falling out. All these weird things were happening, and my GP [general practitioner] at the time tried to tell me that I was just depressed. Luckily, I was seeing a psychiatrist at the time for anxiety, and she was like, "I don't think you're depressed. This is really weird, and you've tried antidepressants in the past, and they always make you manic. So I really don't think depression is what's going on."

She went on, "I usually will have had another doctor who can advocate for me, like my psychiatrist who called my GP saying, 'You need to test her thyroid. I think there's something wrong with her.' So it's not like I had to convince my GP myself."

Relatedly, Ella uses ancestors and living family members' medical histories—elsewhere in space and time, materialized in the clinical appointment via their health stories—to substantiate her claims to physical ailments: "Bringing up, um, family history, I have found helpful; that's also a way I've gotten doctors to do tests that they didn't want to normally do. I've said, 'Well, I've got two aunts and a first cousin, all on the same side of my family, that's got this and now I have the symptoms. Why can't we rule it out?'"

Prior to diagnostic laparoscopy, Beatrice also found it difficult to get diagnostic tests. However, after a surgeon confirmed her severe endometriosis, her credibility as a patient in need of medical care and diagnostic tests improved. As she put it, "Then I can just say I have proof, I officially have stage 3 endo, it's not in my head, and then they're like, 'Oh, okay!' Then the tests were a lot easier to get." The surgeon's credibility, borne out in documentation, bolsters her *ethos*.

Nora, too, relied on printed test results to provide credibility:

> I have found that what I literally have to do, because I was never one that used the patient portal information places to review my medical histories—I found out that I literally have to go onto my portal, print out my results, and take them with me to the doctors. Because I'm finding that there are things, even in the report, it'll specifically say something, and the doctors will look at me and say, "Oh, the report was fine."[18]

In these examples, participants used the credibility proxy—a physically present person, an absent ancestor or living family member, another provider, or a paper trail suggestive of another clinician's opinion or findings—to undo some of the damage done to their credibility by demographic biases and the diagnosis of symptoms as "in their heads." This tactic works since it also helps patients' confidence such that their rhetorical performances are at their best. As Ariana put it, "It's reassuring, in that situation, to have that person in your corner."

Of course, however, the credibility proxy likely works both ways. If a person with stronger *ethos* reifies the "all in your head" assessment, damage can be done. This happened to Leah when, as she recalled, a doctor

doubted the seriousness of her back issues, which ended up requiring surgery. Leah explained that one care provider "admitted he had been influenced by the referring doctor's attitude that there was nothing wrong
with [her]." Other interviewees reported similar frustration with being
unable to shake the stigma that came with a care provider's assessment of
symptoms as psychogenic. As Esther shared, the care provider she went
to for a second opinion was also influenced by her previous care provider's assessment:

> He was reviewing my files, and he started treating me the same way,
> kind of, "Why are you here?" you know, "Did you follow the diet
> plan? . . . In your file, it says you're hysterical and that your opinion
> should be taken with a grain of salt."

While not a common trend in the data, these two strong examples are
worth pointing out as they offer a significant counter-story to successes
with increasing credibility via a third party—a tactic that can easily be
reversed with the wrong proxy.

Emphasizing Day-to-Day Impairment

The credibility proxy, of course, is an acute fix and must, eventually, be
replaced by the patient becoming empowered to offer a complete portrait
of everyday impairment and symptoms. One reason participants gave
for how emphasizing day-to-day impairment was related to their credibility was that it helped to build empathy such that care providers saw
them not only as patients, but as human beings trying to live their lives
and to fulfill their various everyday tasks and obligations. Young and
Flower (2002) helpfully broke down scholarship on theories and practices of patient-provider communication into three categories: "Communication competence among medical professionals"; "Patient-centered
interviewing"; and "The incorporation of empathy-building strategies
into the medical school curriculum" (p. 71). Patients in other studies,
too, have "consistently identified empathy as key to any efficacious clinical encounter" (Kornelsen et al., 2016, p. 374). I coded 53 instances of
participants explaining how they emphasize day-to-day impairment to
bolster credibility, in 28 interviews.

Participants emphasized day-to-day impairment in the hopes of engendering empathy in their care providers such that the seriousness of symptoms would be considered. As one participant, Grace, put it, to get care
providers to take her symptoms seriously: "I kind of have to outright
present it as it is, and kind of have to draw a picture for them and put
them in my shoes." Eliana, too, told her care providers: "I got honors
in my college courses and did very well in my job. I got a promotion
and was highly functional" but, after symptoms came on, she told them,

"I couldn't go anywhere or drive any further than 30 minutes prior to that surgery because of the bowel issues." That is, rather than simply say that she had distressing digestive symptoms, she emphasized the kinds of everyday things she could no longer do—a move that helped to humanize her and to qualify her suffering.

Participants made it clear, though, that this tactic means tailoring the content to what they can ascertain as the physician's value systems. As Lillian explained:

> So for example, my shoulders hurt a lot, so I don't do my hair as much. I put it in a ponytail because it hurts to straighten my hair. My shoulders get stiff. If I explain it that way, it's more relatable because somebody can picture themselves like, "Oh yeah, I guess that could hurt!" I think it's easier to put yourself in a situation, like, "Wow, I can't imagine not straightening my hair," for a female doctor. For a male, it would have to be something else, but situational.

Interestingly, while her male doctor seemed to ignore other descriptions of distress, another participant, Stephanie, eventually had the insight that he would be empathetic, unfortunately, to her husband's plight, noting: "I said to him, 'Look,' and it got his attention, and he looked at me, and I said, 'Look, my sex life is zero. I don't want my husband to leave me.' And he looked up and said, 'Well, we must address that, mustn't we?'"

Chloe also relied on emphasizing impairment over simply naming symptoms: "I have this pain on my left knee, so I just tell them, you know, 'I'm okay when I'm sitting down or when I'm standing up. However, when I try to climb the stairs, I have problems putting weight on my left knee.'" This method paints a picture of everyday impairment such that the care provider can envision themselves or their loved ones similarly incapacitated and might be, thus, more inclined to believe the symptoms are serious signs of a physical problem.

Nina, too, had to stop "kind of doing things outside of school," and she relayed that to her doctor to get approval for an MRI.

When this tactic doesn't work, though, patients' feelings of alienation from care providers increase. Karen recalled her dismay at a doctor in an emergency room who'd dismissed her severe pain with the brush-off, "Did you try an Advil?" As she explained, "Especially, you know, he was a parent, and he should be able to . . . put himself into the position of what amount of pain would cause you to take your two—they were five and under—children to the emergency room at four o'clock in the morning." Still, in many cases, emphasizing day-to-day impairment in descriptive or narrative form, beyond inspiring empathy, also helped participants to demonstrate that symptoms could not be simply "in their heads"; they helped to show that the participants are aware of their bodies' cues and, thus, are in tune with whether they are physically or mentally sick or well. These appeals to *ethos* helped to show that they are capable of reliable self-observation.

Rosa explained the need to be specific thus:

> I think it's really important to try and give enough kind of specific information when I go into an appointment, because I think that can be really helpful to the provider. And I think it also tells them that, okay, so this is somebody who is in tune with their body and knows that something is not right. And I think it also lets them know that, okay, they are really serious about trying to get better or solve the problem, because look at all of the specific information that they were able to provide.

Esther similarly shared details of the fainting she'd experienced to emphasize that she was never feeling stress or anxiety when it came on: "The attacks would happen—there was one that I had at work where—I actually loved my job . . . I had one when I was watching TV, one when I was sitting on the quad, so, there was really nothing that seemed to be in my head about it at all."

Ava used a metaphor to emphasize her level of impairment and self-knowledge following two days of agonizing symptoms that were misattributed to the flu. As she told her care provider, "Look. I need you to listen to me . . . This is how I'm going to explain it. You know when you drive a car, and it's your car, and you've had it for a while. You know if something's wrong with it. If it starts making a different sound, or if it starts acting differently. Well, I know the same thing about my body." Reporting on the success of the metaphor, she shared, "And that's how I got him to listen to me."

Participants also emphasized the day-to-day suffering they experienced to argue for the need to make an ostensibly drastic care decision. They wanted to be clear that they were far from, say, someone with Munchausen syndrome who pathologically seeks out opportunities to be a patient so that they might be on the receiving end of unnecessary medical care and be the recipients of attention and sympathy. Laurine, to illustrate, described her decision to seek excision surgery for endometriosis after her care provider urged her to "exhaust all other options." To persuade him to agree to surgery, she had to tell her doctor: "This is now impeding my daily normal living."

Brenda also commented: "I was beginning to accept that daily pain wasn't normal and it took me a while to just get to that point, just to even say it."

Much like technical diagnostic and laboratory documents stood in for the credibility proxy, some participants kept detailed symptoms journals to provide evidence of day-to-day impairment. These journals documented the temporal details of day-to-day life as it is demoralizingly altered by intrusive, chronic symptoms. Importantly, Schroeder et al. (2017) examined the use of patient-generated data in the form of food and symptoms journals to suggest that diagnosis and treatment plans could be collaboratively reached via this data. My participants expressed a willingness to generate such data.

Acknowledging Care Providers' Expertise and Using Strategic Hedging

Clearly, assigning a credibility proxy and pandering to care providers' ideas of what constitutes significant day-to-day impairment are daunting tactics that participants reluctantly took on because they were pushed to places of desperation and were sincerely and justifiably worried about their lives. In this way, patients in serious need of medical care who've been told they are truly in need of psychiatric care or simple self-care resort to altering their care providers' perceptions of them as the "worried well" and as "hysterical" people relying on inaccurate sources by conveying respect and acceptance of care providers' expertise. Entrepreneur and activist Jackie Carter recently launched a similarly fraught solution to police violence against black men and women during traffic stops with her "Not Reaching pouch"—a transparent pouch that affixes to a dashboard where a driver can store documents commonly requested in a traffic stop such that their movements to obtain these items will not be misread as "reaching" for a weapon (Willingham, 2019, n.p.). Clearly, there is need for continued activism and much more anti-racist work to address the actual issues leading black people to be especially vulnerable to wrongful death in routine circumstances. Still, Carter's pouches solution is an eloquent response to a life or death matter, and some forms of clinical performances are similarly simultaneously dismaying and persuasive solutions to thorny rhetorical problems.

Phillips (2012) argued that "the ways marginalized groups resist the status quo while operating within the status quo should be well considered when analyzing from the vernacular perspective" (p. 263). This notion of "resisting" while "operating within" a biomedical status quo emerged in the data in the form of strategic acknowledgements of care providers' expertise. Likewise, my participants used qualifiers and hedges, such as words or phrases meant to signal uncertainty and tentativeness, to operate within, while tacitly critiquing, the ideological framework that would posit the doctor as expert and the patient as nonexpert. That is, they found that creating effective *ethos* in clinical settings once their symptoms were doubted unfortunately meant pandering to uneven power dynamics with which they do not necessarily agree. However, they saw a need to craft an *ethos* that would fit with the care provider's vision of an ideal (or at least a "good") patient so that they could access better care. Some participants navigated the task of crafting such an *ethos* by consulting their advocacy networks to learn more about how others had managed such performances. That said, they were painfully aware of this rhetorical practice as far from ideal. Indeed, it appears to be an *ethos* to which one might resort if all else seems to be failing and the stakes are incredibly high, such as in contexts in which there is a real fear of increasingly serious morbidity or mortality. I coded 41 instances of this phenomenon in 24 interviews. Gretchen explains the ambivalence with which participants resorted to this tactic (as well as the tactic itself) well:

> So what I do now, which is very sad for me, I had deferred to the doctors. I ask them questions I already know the answers to so that they can build up their ego a little bit. I let them patronize me and laugh at me a little bit. I laugh at myself, and once I get them comfortable with themselves and their own knowledge and own experience, then I will suggest the things that I have found and won't say I have found them.

For many participants, acknowledgements of doctors' expertise allow them to effectively introduce their own research into the clinical scene. Importantly, at times, participants' fears of offending their care providers and, thus, deteriorating relationships, lead them to avoid bringing their high-quality research directly into their appointments, as with Ella, who explained:

> I have an appointment with my endocrinologist that I would like to bring some research in, and I'm questioning whether or not to do it, but just for that reason I don't. He's a great endocrinologist, but my disease is rare, and, you know, I don't see the harm in bringing in credible research, but I also don't want to break down the relationship I have with him, in any way, because he thinks I'm second-guessing him or something.

In this way, they've resorted to strategic apophasis (to say no) or even paralipsis (omission) by learning what *not* to say in an appointment. Keller (2008) called apophasis "the speech of unsaying" to emphasize that the term refers to the strategic mention of an issue or topic in a way that claims to not address that entity (p. 909). Similarly, at times, the tactic of tacitly or overtly acknowledging care providers' expertise is related to pushing for further inquiry into symptoms. Lorna described it as "a lot of ego massaging." When she goes to a care provider to look into a symptom that is being dismissed, she's found it effective to say, "I understand that you're very talented. I'm not questioning your judgment. I am concerned about this and how it impacts me." In this way, she performs a traditional doctor-patient relationship in terms of power via apophasis.

Other participants used something similar to paralipsis, or "a rhetorical device by which a speaker draws attention to an idea that he pretends to pass over" (Crosby, 2013, p. 121).

Gretchen, for example, described how she used her knowledge of upper endoscopy to measure motility thus: "So, instead of saying, 'Can you order me a gastric emptying study,' I said, 'Is there a test? Maybe you know this. I don't know this. But, is there a test that can measure how quickly the stomach empties?'" Gretchen is clear that, while "terrible," this tactic is highly effective. Avery feels similarly: "If they don't really take it seriously when you do your own research, it's kind of like you have to tiptoe around it to lead them to the answer, you know? And that's really terrible."

Also explaining how this tactic relates to the careful presentation of research, Rita explained that she will say to her care provider: "I defer to your judgment, and, you know, your expertise," a position that "seemed to really make a world of difference" in terms of her care provider's willingness to take her seriously.

Nia was also eloquent in her explanation of using this tactic: "It's hard because there's this fine line I feel that you have to walk between being a well-informed patient and overstepping a boundary that doctors don't want you to overstep. That's why I'll be kind of vague because it's hard . . . I have to tone it down and make sure that I'm being the patient." Nia, thus, performs a "good" and compliant patient *ethos*.

Eliana similarly described how she is careful to convey the results of her research in ways that will not appear to disrupt the doctor-patient knowledge hierarchy. As she described her nuanced approach:

> I try not to say "researched something" because they will automatically shut down . . . What I do is pick away the information that has given me my answers, and I present them to the doctors . . . I try to make it where they are the ones telling me and I'm not telling them. Like I tell them my symptoms and just lead them to what I know the answer is.

Commenting on her use of this tactic, too, Stephanie explained how her "willingness to work with the doctors" is what "establishes [her] credibility."

Gretchen summed up this feature of the data quite eloquently:

> I found that works, that doesn't make me feel very good, but it convinces doctors to help me is to play into the dynamic of the power differential between doctor and patient. To ask questions that you already know the answer, to fluff up their ego a little bit, and let them find what you suggest. To ask questions that get them to suggest the things that I want to ask for directly.

In most cases, too, participants are most certainly "performing" this inquisitive and acquiescent patient *ethos* such that the care provider shifts their perception of the patient from mentally unstable and exaggerating, or inventing symptoms to fit internet diagnoses, to a person willing to accept doctor expertise. These performances, while they rarely were self-affirming, were effective.

Performing Symptoms and Demonstrating Illness Severity

Nouri and Rudd asserted that "efforts should be made by providers to reduce oral literacy demand, use plain language, and incorporate the teach-back method, and thereby make conversation more effective and patient-friendly" (p. 570). In some ways, these participants have developed a related way of communicating with providers. Of course, once a person has argued effectively for a specific diagnostic test that they've learned about via research and networking, the physical evidence of disease provides a sizable upshot to *ethos*. Many reported that, once diagnosed with their true afflictions, they went from being treated as emotionally unstable annoyances to serious patients in need of high levels of empathy, compassion, and care. This theme—that once a diagnosis is reached, the person is taken much more seriously, is quite prevalent in the data. This is why diagnosis—an imperfect process that needs a lot more interrogating—is important. Even though, as Teston (2017) eloquently demonstrated in her study of the manufacturing of medical evidence in cancer care, bodies are incredibly homogenous and constantly in flux, and diagnoses themselves are shifting social constructions, diagnoses are immensely powerful ones in terms of credibility in care settings. When participants resorted to performing symptoms, they sought out or stumbled into ways to produce the closest thing possible to objective, empirical evidence of their physical distress. I coded 45 instances of performing symptoms in 23 interviews.

Like others, Laurine's symptoms performance was unintentional, yet quite effective. During a pelvic exam, she literally lost consciousness—a symptom she'd been unsuccessfully emphasizing as a clear sign of a serious physical problem. Her reports of fainting, though, were perhaps read as exaggerations, since a care provider took it much more seriously after witnessing the event in a clinical appointment in real time. As she put it, "When I finally came to, I'm like, 'This is the best day ever because you finally, like, someone, I'm not making this up.'"

Samuel similarly stumbled into a symptoms performance quite by accident. Having trouble explaining episodes of involuntary movement and mild aphasia, Samuel was able to get a diagnosis, in part, by performing the symptom: "He was checking my stomach, and something that he pressed. He pressed on my stomach, and I just started wigging out. He got to see it."

Others appeared in clinical appointments with dramatic weight loss, such as Melissa who ended up "getting down to 70-something pounds." In the same way, after Amelia's doctor indicated that he believed her numbness was weight related, she returned having "lost 75 pounds" with no improvement in her numbness. Grace similarly found that it took her getting "so weak and fragile for them to say, 'Okay, maybe this isn't in your head.'"

Mila explained the dangers of failing to perform distress, recalling, "The nurse comes in and says, 'I thought I would find you writhing in pain.' And I said, 'This is how I writhe.' I think people don't pay attention because I'm not demonstrative enough. You know what I mean?"

Lucy similarly explained how an autoimmune flare can subside by the time a person reaches an appointment date, which can make it difficult to convey the severity of the symptoms that were worse and could return. She explained, "I wasn't actively having a whole lot of symptoms, they were tampering off," and this reality made the appointment more challenging.

Some forms of bodily performance, though, were not helpful in terms of bolstering credibility. Many reported that crying or avoiding eye contact hurts credibility and made a diagnosis of anxiety and an attendant dismissal of all symptoms as related to that diagnosis more likely. Trying to appear calm, then, is very much a part of clinical performance.

Advocate (Repositioning the Self in Relation to Health Outcomes)

While clinical performances could be happy ephemeral accidents that led to strong *ethos*, adapting a self-advocate *ethos* was quite purposeful. Participants in this study indicated that they had to become their own advocates to get better care and to, thus, gain more favorable health outcomes. In fact, the word "advocate" appears 62 times in 31 of the 68 interviews coded, and the specific phrase "become my own advocate" appears 54 times in 28 of the interviews. Further investigation revealed that participants referred to themselves as having become their own advocates when they put in the time to determine the kind of care to which they were entitled and made specific, strategic, and proactive steps and requests to gain better care; put simply, they asked for what they needed in a direct manner. They performed as their "own advocate" by speaking up and being specific about what they expected from their clinical appointments. More than performing as advocates, though, this positioning of themselves as self-advocates—calling themselves that and understanding themselves as such—changed their behaviors in ways that bolstered their *ethos*. Once they adjusted their subject positions from passive patient to active self-advocate, they began to seek out ways to collaborate with their care providers to find answers to and relief from confounding symptoms. When they did not get the care they knew they needed, they sought out new care providers.

Position Self as Own Advocate

Annie explained how her willingness to position herself as her own advocate helped her to avoid being denied treatment for an *E. coli* infection:

> I was in law school, and I was very sick and with, you know, diarrhea and vomiting and all other terrible symptoms. I had gone to the doctor, and they were saying, "Oh, your symptoms, the way you are describing them, the timing doesn't make sense." And so I actually had to insist, like, "Well I want you to do this and send a sample," and then turns out I had *E. coli.*

In sharp contrast to acknowledging care providers' expertise, and beyond preparing and performing successful appeals to *ethos*, then, participants' journeys to appropriate care relied on their taking on self-advocate positions. More than merely performing as advocates, though, participants learned to internalize the idea that they themselves were in the best position to push for the best care—a shift in sense of self that led to stronger performances of *ethos*. Often, participants used language related to force, such as "pushing" or "fighting" or "demanding" to describe their self-advocacy, as in Glynis, for example, who described: "I come in armed with papers from academic journals, with a list of questions to say, 'This is what I need,'—advocating for myself."

Lillian as well explained, "From there, I really kept pushing that something was wrong and so she finally listened to me." Luna also explained how repositioning herself as her own advocate changed the tenor of her care: "I am assertive, I tell them what's going on, I can call them, I can say, 'No, this isn't right,' and they believe me and they follow through with it."

Grace explained advocacy as synonymous with proactive decision-making:

> That's what I advocate for is, the doctors come in, they kind of explain what's going on in layman's terms, and your treatment, and you've got to weigh the pros and cons of that medication. And you can refuse to take it if you want, or you can take it and see how you do.

Reflecting on her journey to becoming a self-advocate, Riley explained:

> I feel like the doctors listen to me now because I demand that. Initially, the first five, six, seven years, I was just in the middle of confusion and not understanding what was going on. After so much time of living with the illness, I feel like I have the control to get the doctors to help me.

Nina also asserted, "I have to be the best advocate for myself." Maggie slated her own advocacy statement as advice for others: "Don't be afraid to stick up for yourself and be your own advocate. It's always worth it. You're worth it." Rosa noted that it's "not always comfortable" yet one must be "willing to speak up." Mila described a successful medical appointment after she'd been dismissed as wearing her "big guns that day" and refusing to leave until she got attention and care. Mia recalled how becoming her own advocate involved directing her care team via electronic tools: "So I have a patient portal set up. So I send a message to, like one doctor, but I cc all my other doctors." Roundtree, Dorsten, and Reif (2011) posited that "work on the development of new communication technologies (e.g. Web 2.0, social media, and web-based platforms for the development of lifestyle change) from rhetorical and communication theory perspectives can provide important insights to clinicians, medical researchers, and the institutions involved in disseminating their findings" and that "the theory and practice of communication is directly tied to the success and implementation of new technology" (p. 8). Mia's comments hint at these realities.

These forms of advocacy mirror tropes of the medical-establishment-resistance narrative, but also showcase patients' moves to shift power dynamics such that they are collaborators in their own care and that they are willing to let go of the notion that illnesses have linear progressions.

Collaborate With Care Providers

Moss, Reiter, Rimer, and Brewer (2016) found that collaborative patient-provider communication that was "provider driven" yet "shared and efficient" led to higher levels of uptake of teen vaccinations (p. 106). Young and Flower (2002) offer a rhetorical model of healthcare communication that positions the patient as problem-solver and decision-maker" (p. 71) They advocate for a "collaborative interpretation" toward a "shared pool of information" (p. 86). Relatedly, in contrast to the last-ditch performative efforts at establishing a "good patient" *ethos*, participants have sometimes managed to reframe care providers' expertise as a way to facilitate effective collaborative conversations. They've done so by reminding their care providers that while doctors have a lot of expertise, they do not and cannot know everything. Pointing out this logic challenges some basic epistemologies at work when care providers give patients definitive diagnoses of psychogenic symptoms when such assessments can never be certain.

When participants positioned themselves as their own advocates, they often also attempted to shift the tenor of the relationship such that they took on an *ethos* of knowledgeable collaborator in their care. Importantly, "when illness is fraught with uncertainty, this therapeutic relationship becomes paramount." (Kornelsen et al., 2016, p. 374). Many participants found that they had more credibility in clinical encounters when they put forth a good amount of effort to establish an "honest, empathetic, and enduring relationship" with their care providers such that the spaces of time in which no diagnosis was present could be marked not by suspicion and accusation of mental health issues, but by "a shared intimacy and acceptance of uncertainty" (Kornelsen et al., 2016, p. 374). I coded 43 instances of participants managing to collaborate with care providers in 20 interviews.

Riley, for instance, made it clear, as did others, that reaching a place where this level of collaboration is possible takes time, as one must establish a strong *ethos* to arrive at that place. "I've been seeing him since 2005, so over time our relationship has changed," she explained of her own care provider. "At first," she continued, "I would go in and just be kind of the student sitting there. Whatever he told me to do, I did. Now, I feel like, I come in and I kind of tell him, this is what's going on, this is what I think we should do. Ninety percent of the time, that's what he does."

Grace has also become successful using her position as self-advocate and informed patient to assert herself as a viable collaborator in her own care, noting:

> They said, "Now it's spread to all four lobes of your lung," and I looked at them, and I said, "Why don't you do a bronchoscopy?" The doctor looked at me and he said, "You know what? I think we need to do that." . . . I've had to many times say, "Why don't we look at this?" They say, "You know what? That's a great idea."

Interestingly, Nora described how her efforts to position herself as a collaborator with her general care doctor led him to suggest a collaborative experiment that yielded results as described above wherein her doctor put her on a medication to provide evidence that her symptoms were autoimmune-related rather than psychogenic such that the rheumatologist would substantiate that diagnosis.

McKenzie explained the importance of finding a care provider with whom it is possible to collaborate, noting:

> So I think that is the key. To find someone to bounce those ideas off of and it can kind of keep you in check, but it can also be open enough that you both can sit down and figure out what is going on.

Establishing an *ethos* of collaborator in your own care, of course, requires a provider who'll be amenable to this dynamic. As Sandra commented, "I just have been lucky, I guess, in finding doctors who will work with me to figure out what makes me feel normal because I'm very good at just tracking stuff myself and sort of knowing when something's off."

While many were emphatic about "advocacy" as a term that inspired and described making demands and being a proactive participant in one's own care, Sandra paired that emphasis with the need to avoid inappropriate or unnecessary medical interventions by working with the right provider:

> Unless you're seeking out the solution yourself and working with a provider who wants to find you that solution as well, you're not going to get as far as you could, necessarily. I still am amazed that if I had just listened to my gynecologist, she would have been operating on me for no reason.

When such a relationship is impossible to establish, purposefully and proactively seeking out a new care provider can be a way to bolster credibility via proving that the "in your head" diagnosis was incorrect all along. Considering the rhetorical dimensions of the patient-provider encounter, Sharf (1990) argued that effective patient-provider communication in medical interviewing leads to "a narrative co-construction that weaves threads of both points of view into the fabric" (p. 229). Participants also sought out opportunities to establish collaborative relationships via communication.

Seek Out a New Care Provider

A limitation of the advocate *ethos*, of course, is that participants also report that being too forceful or argumentative runs the risk of confirming a provider's assessment of your symptoms being "in your head" and/or of you being mentally unstable. As Luna explained, patients are "disempowered" by the "medical establishment" when they settle for care providers that do not connect them with support networks and provide literature through which patients can learn more about their conditions. In such cases, Luna asserted, moving on to a better provider is key. Importantly, participants relied on social networks and online reviews to identify new care providers, but their ability to see new providers or not naturally had a lot to do with material conditions such as insurance, geographic location, and financial resources. When they were fortunate enough to get a new provider, that person could be key to unlocking the mysteries of their symptoms. I coded 58 instances of participants seeking out new care providers in 32 interviews.

That said, seeking out new care providers can have the unintended effect of lessening credibility. Leah's case illustrates the complexity of seeking out new care providers; she was "accused of doctor shopping." Nonetheless, moving on from care providers who'd doubted her symptoms led to an accurate diagnosis. In an effort to prevent future errors, Leah, a nurse and patient advocate, "sent letters (low key and not accusatory)" to those who'd misdiagnosed her, "pointing out these conditions were quite obvious and quite serious." Even after she was sure to include information indicating that she did not plan to sue, one specialty center's neuro-radiologist got in touch with Leah to ask if she planned to sue. Her response was, "No, but that no one should have missed a spinal condition that severe, that obvious, and that disabling." The care provider, then, as noted above, admitted he had been influenced by the referring doctor's attitude that there was nothing wrong with her and assured her that he would "never make the mistake of assuming the referring doctor's diagnosis was correct without doing his own in-depth review again." Thus, despite that the referring doctor undermined the patient's credibility in this instance, advocacy likely changed the tenor of care for future patients via Leah's measured way of pointing out medical error.

Many participants contemplated the long road to diagnoses and how they wished they'd found new care providers sooner. For instance, Glynis reflected:

> I think people, they go to the doctor's and they feel like, well, I have to see this doctor. I have to see him because this is who I was sent to and I have no other option even though I don't like him. Knowing that you can change, or you have that much power, it helps.

Luna also explained that if a doctor implies that her symptoms are in her head, she takes that as a clear sign that they do not belong on her care team. Irene similarly explained, "If you're not even interested enough to find out why I'm there, I don't see much point in going on."

For many participants, finding care providers that are willing to move beyond obvious diagnoses is key to getting good care when symptoms are wrongly diagnosed as "in your head." As Sandra put it:

> I know on a lot of medical TV shows, they say the expression, "If you hear hoof steps, think horses not zebras." In my experience, I'm always a zebra, and most doctors don't want to see that unless I draw them a map. Or I finally find the doctor who is like, "Yes, actually let's consider that you might not be the easiest answer to this question. You might be the randomest [sic] answer I've ever seen."

Of course, even sharing her familiarity with the horses/zebras saying could be read as an *ethos*-bolstering tactic. As well, choosing new care providers when your symptoms are not believed to be signs of serious physical distress is empowering. As Grace put it:

> For me, to walk out of the doctor's office and feel like I achieved something or we're on the right track, I have to have credibility. If not, I do not go back to that doctor. I divorce them, put it that way.

That said, this approach to self-empowerment assumes that other care providers are available to the patient, and that is clearly not always the case. When a person must continue to work with a care provider, other strategies for repairing damaged *ethos* must be relied upon, and this chapter shares a number of alternative approaches to finding another care provider when such a move is not an option. Chapter 5 similarly uses field-based data collected at an outpatient facility for adults with chronic mental illness diagnoses to theorize everyday strategies for regaining credibility in the context of extreme stigma. Still, when other care providers are an option, choosing a new care provider—particularly when the new provider helps to find physical causes for symptoms—can empower the patient and repair *ethos*.

Conclusion

Among several recommendations for increasing patient engagement and, thus, enhancing patient-provider communication and health outcomes, Jenerette and Mayer (2016) suggested the use of the SBAR (situation, background, assessment, recommendation) method as it "uses a communication syntax familiar to health care providers," so "its use by patients when communicating with health care providers could lead to positive interactions while setting the tone for the remainder of the visit by enhancing credibility, trust, and positive self-presentation" (p. 140). This interview research also suggests ways patients might generate better interactions with providers, but it uses patients' everyday strategies rather than established provider communication practices to build out a framework.

Much like other studies that take up grounded theory methods, this chapter has demonstrated a "commitment to analyzing social processes, using comparative methods, accepting a provisional view of truth, fostering the emergence of new ideas, and providing tools for constructing substantive and formal middle-range theories" (Charmaz & Belgrave, 2015, p. 2). Multipronged approaches to establishing or rebuilding *ethos* are needed in circumstances like the ones many of my participants found themselves in, where symptoms were deemed "in their heads" without any investigation beyond a very brief clinical conversation. As Lorna put it, "I feel like that's the goal of every woman who goes to a doctor, is to be taken seriously." And the same can be said for others with marks of difference. An important caveat to all of the tactics for bolstering credibility described above is that they don't always work for every person in every circumstance. This reality accounts for the fact that some tactics for establishing, repairing, and/or bolstering *ethos* actually contradict others. Considering ephemeral rhetorical moves as tactics everyday rhetors use to bolster their credibility after a stigmatizing misdiagnosis means honoring the inconsistencies and flux that mark their existence. Still, as the data above shows, these individual tactics, even as they emerge in ephemeral clinical encounters that span wide swaths of space and time, have the capacity to become advocacy strategies when sustained, adapted, and supported by others. It is also important to note that misdiagnosis is a common occurrence—even when no biases or stigmas are at play and even when care providers are trying in earnest to get to the bottom of symptoms. After all, bias has influenced medical research, clinical protocols, and a range of other practices that are beyond the scope of this chapter, but are nonetheless important to recognize. Moreover, there are clear cases where mental health struggles do, in fact, lead to physical symptoms; physical struggles, of course, can also lead to mental health issues.

Accurately diagnosing patients with complex and misunderstood physical symptoms—many of whom might have such conditions under the guise of psychogenic diagnoses—is an important step toward more equitable health outcomes. Diagnosis, of course, doesn't always mean a cure or even a treatment plan that will restore functionality. More research of all kinds—including rhetoric of health and medicine research—is needed on many complex conditions, including research that engages providers. Another issue that needs far more research is the reality that some people's pain is simply not taken very seriously. Problematically, that is, credibility is sometimes earned and many times not. As Beatrice reflected, "Unfortunately, some of the credibility I have earned was because of my own privilege."

Kornelsen et al. (2016) argued that "healthcare professionals' commitment to relationships" might be "the potential locus of healing rather than an identified diagnosis or treatment," and they advocate for medical training to include such compassionate care (p. 375). Equally important, though, is the need to train physicians to continue to look for underlying physical causes when perhaps demographic markers hit up against social performances and lead the care provider to hastily reach a diagnosis of medically unexplained physical symptoms or even psychogenic symptoms due to attendant beliefs about the patient's credibility.

Kennedy (2012) wrote convincingly on the "inevitable, negative consequences of fallacious psychogenic explanations" that "cause iatrogenic effects on patients' lives" (p. 219). Gretchen's and Smirl's cases that begin this chapter make it rather unsurprising that even Francis[19] (2013)—a long-time contributor to psychiatric bodies of knowledge—expressed concern with information published by the *Diagnostic and Statistical Manual of Mental Disorders, Fifth Edition* (DSM-V) working group on the diagnostic category "somatic symptom disorder" (SSD). Like other revisions in the DSM-V, this diagnostic group offered broad and inclusive criteria and eliminated diagnoses of somatization disorder, hypochondriasis, pain disorder, and undifferentiated somatoform in favor of a single term. The open-ended nature of this new grouping, lamented Francis, offers practitioners credible ways to diagnose a wide swath of the population with psychological problems when their physical symptoms do not *appear* to have causes. This is a good example of how a tactic can move to an institutionally sanctioned strategy. "A false positive diagnosis of somatic symptom disorder harms patients because it may result in the underlying medical causes being missed. It also subjects patients to stigma, inappropriate drugs, psychotherapy, and iatrogenic disease," (p. 26) Francis opined.

This shortcoming was likely not the intention of the working group charged with rewriting this category's diagnostic criteria. Quite the opposite—the new language was a clear attempt to mitigate the possibility of misdiagnosing an organic disease as a psychiatric problem by eliminating the diagnostic criterion that said a patient should have no known physical illness to qualify as having a somatic condition. However, it is clear that the new criteria, ironically, make it possible to diagnose more patients with SSD. Naturally, the confusion over how to treat physical symptoms without known organic causes perplexes physicians who must contend with how to name the unknown and to avoid offending their patients (Ding & Kanaan, 2016). However, attempts to make diagnosis more precise and to cut down on misdiagnosis, paradoxically, in practice, led to discursive constructions that make it easier to diagnose more people than ever.

For the misdiagnosed and undiagnosed—especially those with increasingly problematic symptoms that significantly deplete quality of life and interfere with day-to-day function, a diagnosis can be incredibly relieving. Even in cases where treatment options are few, the symbolic meaning of the diagnosis itself is a powerful boost to a person's sense of self-worth as it verifies the physical cause of the symptoms and dismantles the fiction that they are suffering from mental health problems alone.

In a related way, comorbidity complicates credibility—particularly when a person has a mental health diagnosis they agree with, but the new symptoms are not manifestations of that condition. This chapter has shown the repercussions of this misattribution of mental health causes for medical disease symptoms. The potential for missed opportunities to effectively treat physical health problems multiplies when a long history of mental illness diagnosis is also present. Thus, research is needed to learn more on how those with serious mental health diagnoses argue effectively for their credibility following highly stigmatizing experiences. Such is the focus of Chapter 5.

Notes

1. Gretchen is a pseudonym as are all other names of participants, care providers, and hospitals.
2. This research was approved by James Madison University's institutional review board on March 21, 2017, ID Number 17–0412.

3. Dauntingly, it should be noted that Gretchen's road to diagnosis was quite short—even at two years—compared to other participants, some of whom navigated inaccurate psychogenic-symptoms diagnoses for well over a decade.

4. An explanation of how I developed codes can be found in the "Participant Recruitment, Methods, Limitations" section of this chapter.

5. I also use Smirl's case in a chapter that will be in Frost and Eble's forthcoming edited volume *Interrogating Gendered Pathologies.*

6. Psychogenic diagnoses are given when care providers believe that physical symptoms arise from mental or emotional distress and/or mental illness rather than from physical disease or illness.

7. Not all instances of medically unexplained physical symptoms (MUPS), of course, are due to misdiagnosis. Indeed, "when common diagnoses are exhausted, physicians will turn to investigating less common possibilities," and "at the moment of perceived saturation where all known diagnostic possibilities have been excluded, physicians—and patients—confront uncertainty in diagnosis" (Kornelsen, Atkins, Brownell, & Woollard, 2016, p. 367).

8. It should be noted that two of the 68 people interviewed still do not have a diagnosis of physical disease.

9. As I explain elsewhere (Molloy, 2019), "Snowball sampling is a common nonprobability sampling method used for qualitative research projects. Snowball sampling is a useful method when the target population is difficult to identify or reach; like other nonprobability sampling methods, it is appropriate when a potential population is almost limitless due to the fact that whether a person fits inclusion criteria is impossible to predict in advance. In the Credibility at the Clinic study, for example, it was not possible to clearly identify the subset of the population who had experiences with misdiagnoses of psychogenic symptoms without casting a wide net and asking a large group of people to identify whether they had that experience."

10. Surveys were fully anonymous, but they ended with a link to a nonanonymous survey through which participants could indicate their willingness to be contacted for a follow-up interview. I was fortunate enough to collect 1414 survey responses over the course of recruiting participants for this study. Importantly, the survey data contains narrative questions that are very similar to interview questions, and responses confirm the coding scheme developed for analyses of interview data. That said, due to scope, the survey data is not cited in this chapter.

11. I do not name the organizations and groups I was fortunate enough to work with for participant recruitment, as a measure to further protect participant anonymity.

12. Of course, interview questions did not explicitly ask for participants to disclose demographic information. However, data on race, age, gender, and social class emerged explicitly and implicitly during interviews during participants' responses to other questions.

13. While I agree with Dubriwny's (2013) critique of the trope of the "the vulnerable empowered woman" and its reliance on women becoming empowered "through the act of choice, framed in terms of consumption of medical treatments, diagnostic tests, and products such as red dress pins" (Dubriwny, 2013, p. 8), the women and men in my study relied on diagnostic tests and their results to move past assumed psychogenic symptoms and toward appropriate treatment.

14. I also coded for misdiagnosis, symptoms labelled "all in the person's head," judgments that symptoms were manifestations of mental health problems, and biases and judgments. These issues are found in Chapter 2.

15. Readers will note that "self-doctoring" often refers to doctors inappropriately treating themselves for medical conditions (see, for example, Fromme,

Hebert, & Carrese, 2004), but Emmons (2010) uses the term to mean patients acting as their own doctors.
16. Collecting and analyzing such texts would have been quite advantageous, yet such practices were not part of the study design. Still, including these texts in future studies would be generative.
17. It is important to note that while the majority of my interviewees were women, the men in the study who'd experienced misdiagnosis and delayed diagnosis employed similar strategies to build their credibility. A larger study might note differences between genders.
18. Here, readers will note that the participant needed to acquire the literacies necessary to read her own test results. She had to do high-quality textual research. This is an example of how these strategies inevitably layer and stack.
19. It should also be noted, however, that Francis is a frequent critic of DSM-V and of excesses in psychiatry that lead to overtreatment/overdiagnosis.

References

Batterham, R. W., Hawkins, M., Collins, P. A., Buchbinder, R., & Osborne, R. H. (2016). Health literacy: Applying current concepts to improve health services and reduce health inequalities. *Public Health*, *132*, 3–12. doi:10.1016/j.puhe.2016.01.001.

Bennett, J. (2014). *Born this way: Queer vernacular and the politics of origins* Routledge. doi:10.1080/14791420.2014.924153.

Castro, Y., Carbonell, J. L., & Anestis, J. C. (2012). The influence of gender role on the prediction of antisocial behaviour and somatization. *The International Journal of Social Psychiatry*, *58*(4), 409–416. doi:10.1177/0020764011406807.

Chapman, E. N., Kaatz, A., & Carnes, M. (2013). Physicians and implicit bias: How doctors may unwittingly perpetuate healthcare disparities. *Journal of General Internal Medicine*, *28*(11), 1504–1510. doi:10.1007/s11606-013-2441-1.

Charmaz, K., & Belgrave, L. L. (2015). Grounded theory. In *The Blackwell Encyclopedia of Sociology*, G. Ritzer (Ed.). doi:10.1002/9781405165518.wbeosg070.pub2.

Crosby, R. B. (2013). Mitt Romney's Paralipsis: (Un)veiling Jesus in "Faith in America." *Rhetoric Review*, *32*(2), 119–136.

Derkatch, C. (2016). *Bounding biomedicine: Evidence and rhetoric in the new science of alternative medicine*. Chicago, IL: University of Chicago Press.

Ding, J. M., & Kanaan, R. A. A. (2016). What should we say to patients with unexplained neurological symptoms? How explanation affects offence. *Journal of Psychosomatic Research*, *91*, 55–60. doi:10.1016/j.jpsychores.2016.10.012.

Dryden, L. (Producer), & Brea, J. (Director). (2017). Unrest. [Video/DVD] Shella Films. Retrieved from www.imdb.com/title/tt3268850/

Dubriwny, T. (2013). *The vulnerable empowered woman: Feminism, postfeminism, and women's health*. New Brunswick, NJ: Rutgers University Press.

Duff, L. (2012). And now some words from my friends: Lisa. Retrieved from https://outlivinglungcancer.com/2012/11/18/and-now-some-words-from-my-friends-lisa/

Dusenbery, M. (2018a). *Doing harm: The truth about how bad medicine and lazy science leave women dismissed, misdiagnosed, and sick*. New York: HarperCollins.

Dusenbery, M. (2018b). Everybody was telling me there was nothing wrong. Retrieved from www.bbc.com/future/story/20180523-how-gender-bias-affects-your-healthcare

Elo, S., Kääriäinen, M., Isola, A., & Kyngäs, H. (2013). Developing and testing a middle-range theory of the well-being supportive physical environment of home-dwelling elderly. *The Scientific World Journal, 2013*, 945635. doi:10.1155/2013/945635.

Emmons, K. (2010). *Black dogs and blue words: Depression and gender in the age of self-care*. New Brunswick, NJ: Rutgers University Press.

Endres, D., Hess, A., Senda-Cook, S., & Middleton, M. K. (2016). In situ rhetoric. *Cultural Studies, Critical Methodologies, 16*(6), 511–524. doi:10.1177/1532708616655820.

Fowler, D. (2018, October 29). Women share all the times their medical problems were ignored by doctors. Yahoo Finance Retrieved from https://finance.yahoo.com/news/women-share-personal-stories-medical-problems-ignored-twitter-140705603.html

Francis, A. (2013). *Saving normal: An insider's revolt against out-of-control psychiatric diagnosis, DSM-5, big pharma, and the medicalization of ordinary life*. New York: Harper Collins.

Fromme, E. K., Hebert, R. S., & Carrese, J. A. (2004). Self-doctoring: A qualitative study of physicians with cancer. *The Journal of Family Practice, 53*(4) Retrieved from www.mdedge.com/familymedicine/article/60225/self-doctoring-qualitative-study-physicians-cancer

Graham, S. S. (2015). *The politics of pain medicine: A rhetorical-ontological inquiry*. Chicago, IL: University of Chicago Press.

Hernández, L. H., & Dean, M. (2019). "I felt very discounted": Negotiation of Caucasian and Hispanic/Latina women's bodily ownership and expertise in patient-provider interactions. In E. Frost & M. Eble (Eds.), *Interrogating gendered pathologies* (n.p). Louisville, CO: Utah State University Press. Forthcoming.

Hess, A. (2011). Critical-rhetorical ethnography: Rethinking the place and process of rhetoric. *Communication Studies, 62*(2), 127–152. doi:10.1080/10510974.2011.529750.

Hoffmann, D. E., & Tarzian, A. J. (2001). The girl who cried pain: A bias against women in the treatment of pain. *Journal of Law, Medicine, and Ethics, 29*, 13–27. doi:10.2139/ssrn.383803.

hooks, b. (1990). *Yearning: Race, gender, and cultural politics*. Boston, MA: South End Press.

Ingraham, C. (2013). Talking (about) the elite and mass: Vernacular rhetoric and discursive status. *Philosophy & Rhetoric, 46*(1), 1–21. doi:10.5325/philrhet.46.1.0001.

Jenerette, C. M., & Mayer, D. K. (2016). Patient-provider communication: The rise of patient engagement. *Seminars in Oncology Nursing, 32*(2), 134–143. doi:10.1016/j.soncn.2016.02.007.

Johnson, J. (2010). The skeleton on the couch: The Eagleton affair, rhetorical disability, and the stigma of mental illness. *Rhetoric Society Quarterly, 40*(5), 459–478. doi:10.1080/02773945.2010.517234.

Kalin, J., & Gruber, D. (2018). Gut rhetorics: Toward experiments in living with microbiota. *Rhetoric of Health & Medicine, 1*(3–4), 269–295. doi:10.5744/rhm.2018.1014.

Keller, C. (2008). The apophasis of gender: A fourfold unsaying of feminist theology. *Journal of the American Academy of Religion, 76*(4), 905–933. doi:10.1093/jaarel/lfn090.

Kennedy, A. (2012). *Authors of our own misfortune?: The problems with psychogenic explanations for physical illnesses*. New York: Village Digital Press.

Kornelsen, J., Atkins, C., Brownell, K., & Woollard, R. (2016). The meaning of patient experiences of medically unexplained physical symptoms. *Qualitative Health Research*, 26(3), 367–376. doi:10.1177/1049732314566326.

Ladwig, K. H., Marten-Mittag, B., Erazo, N., & Gündel, H. (2001). Identifying somatization disorder in a population-based health examination survey: Psychosocial burden and gender differences. *Psychosomatics, 42*(6), 511–518.

Levy, G. (2018, April 20). Dying to be heard. US News and World Report Retrieved from www.usnews.com/news/the-report/articles/2018-04-20/why-women-struggle-to-get-doctors-to-believe-them

Liehr, P., & Smith, M. J. (2017). Middle range theory: A perspective on development and use. ANS *Advances in Nursing Science*, 40(1), 51–63. doi:10.1097/ANS.0000000000000162.

Molloy, C. (2019). Durable, portable research through partnerships with interdisciplinary advocacy groups, specific research topics, and larger data sets. *Technical Communication Quarterly*, 28(2), 165–176. doi:10.1080/10572252.2019.1588375.

Moss, J. L., Reiter, P. L., Rimer, B. K., & Brewer, N. T. (2016). Collaborative patient-provider communication and uptake of adolescent vaccines. *Social Science & Medicine, 159*, 100–107. doi:10.1016/j.socscimed.2016.04.030.

Novella, S. (2009). *It's all in your head*. Retrieved from https://sciencebasedmedicine.org/its-all-in-your-head/

Papillion, T. (1995). Isocrates' techne and rhetorical pedagogy. *Rhetoric Society Quarterly*, 25(1–4), 149–163. doi:10.1080/02773949509391038.

Phillips, J. D. (2012). Engaging men and boys in conversations about gender violence: Voice male magazine using vernacular rhetoric as social resistance. *The Journal of Men's Studies, 20*(3), 259–273. doi:10.3149/jms.2003.259.

Rai, C. (2016). *Democracy's lot: Rhetoric, publics, and the places of invention*. Tuscaloosa, AL: University of Alabama Press.

Roundtree, A., Dorsten, A., & Reif, J. (2011). Improving patient activation in crisis and chronic care through rhetorical approaches to new media technologies. *Poroi, 7*(1). doi:10.13008/2151-2957.1081.

Saldaña, J. (2016). *The coding manual for qualitative researchers* (3rd ed.). Thousand Oaks, CA: Sage Publications.

Schroeder, J., Hoffswell, J., Chung, C., Fogarty, J., Munson, S., & Zia, J. (2017). Supporting patient-provider collaboration to identify individual triggers using food and symptom journals. Paper presented at the 1726–1739. doi:10.1145/2998181.2998276. Retrieved from http://doi.acm.org/10.1145/2998181.2998276

Schwartz, D. D., Stewart, S. D., Aikens, J. E., Bussell, J. K., Osborn, C. Y., & Safford, M. M. (2017). Seeing the person, not the illness: Promoting diabetes medication adherence through patient-centered collaboration. *Clinical Diabetes: A Publication of the American Diabetes Association, 35*(1), 35–42. doi:10.2337/cd16-0007.

Sharf, B. F. (1990). Physician--patient communication as interpersonal rhetoric: A narrative approach. *Health Communication*, 2(4), 217–231. doi:10.1207/s15327027hc0204_2.

Shen, M., Hamann, H., Thomas, A., & Ostroff, J. (2016). Association between patient-provider communication and lung cancer stigma. *Supportive Care in Cancer*, 24(5), 2093–2099. doi:10.1007/s00520-015-3014-0.

Teston, C. (2017). *Bodies in flux: Scientific methods for negotiating medical uncertainty.* Chicago, IL: University of Chicago Press.

Weiss, S. (2018, October 16). Women with chronic illnesses: How long & how many doctors did it take you to get diagnosed?. Retrieved from https://twitter.com/suzannahweiss/status/1052249111225720832?lang=en

White, R. O., Chakkalakal, R. J., Presley, C. A., Bian, A., Schildcrout, J. S., Wallston, K. A., . . . Rothman, R. (2016). Perceptions of provider communication among vulnerable patients with diabetes: Influences of medical mistrust and health literacy. *Journal of Health Communication, 21*(Supp 2), 127–134. doi:10.1080/10810730.2016.1207116.

Willingham, A. J. (2019, April 30). This woman is trying to protect black motorists during traffic stops with one small invention. *CNN.* Retrieved from www.cnn.com/2019/04/30/us/not-reaching-pouch-police-shooting-race-traffic-trnd/index.html

Wool, C., & Barsky, A. (1994). Do women somatize more than men? Gender differences in somatization. *Psychosomatics, 35*(5), 445–452.

Yansá, Y. (2019). Bio of Yamani Yansá. Retrieved from www.yamaniyansa.com/bio

Young, A., & Flower, L. (2002). Patients as partners, patients as problem-solvers. *Health Communication, 14*(1), 69–97. doi:10.1207/S15327027HC1401_4.

4 Phantom Limb Pain and Tacit Appeals to *Ethos*

When Patients' Self-Knowledge Exceeds Existing Clinical Knowledge and Predicts Future Clinical Findings

Introduction

Phantom limb pain (PLP), which is quite common in amputees, is the feeling that the missing limb is present, but paralyzed and/or painfully contorted (Kim & Kim, 2012; Ramachandran & Rogers-Ramachandran, 1996). Researchers agree that, while it is not always acknowledged as such, PLP is a significant issue due to its severity, its chronic nature, and its relation to lower quality of life and functionality for patients (Collins et al., 2018). In the archival data used as evidence in this chapter, US Civil War veteran Lewis Atherton explained his PLP in response to a survey mailed to him decades after his injury. This survey was meant to collect data on "remote consequences" of wartime limb loss (Mitchell, 1895).

"It gives me no peace," Atherton wrote. His statement, read over a hundred years later, could easily have been written by today's amputees who also find PLP to be a chronic and even debilitating condition. In fact, researchers who've worked with amputees still identify PLP—a nagging and ever-present source of discomfort—as one of the most significant detriments to post-amputation quality of life (van der Schans, Geertzen, Schoppen, & Dijkstra, 2002). When another veteran Chat K. Ritchey described his PLP as part of the same 19th century research, he made it clear, in a letter he sent along with his completed survey, that he believed that the research could bring relief in his lifetime. As he put it:

> My suffering has been severe at times in my feet that are gone sometimes both and other only one. I call it double geared lightning. It is so severe they are the worst at night. I shall hope that you will find the causes and also be able to furnish us some relief. I shall hope to hear from you again.
>
> (n.p.)

These surveys—remarkably modern qualitative health research tools—align powerfully with the themes of this book since, as I'll describe below, they contain everyday appeals to *ethos* that are in response to stigmatizing experiences related to a confounding health condition—one with uncertain etiologies. They also bring an important element to the collective project of this book by calling attention to the prescience and intelligence of participants' vernacular descriptions of their own bodies and minds. In the participants' words, etched in fading pen and pencil on blue cardstock, there are reminders of how qualitative health research is often inadequately reciprocal for participants and how the data is likely always more valuable than the projects can bear out. Thus, data in these surveys illustrates the significance of building adaptable theories from participants' everyday contributions such that their impact is greater—a move that honors their gifts. Unearthing these surveys, bringing them out of the archives and into a contemporary analysis in a book alongside contemporary data, posthumously ennobles these participants' contributions by showing that while the research in which they took part did not solve the mysteries of PLP, a contemporary examination of their words shows that the data to which they generously contributed did contain seeds from which contemporary findings might have been drawn.

This chapter, thus, also argues that looking back on and re-examining qualitative health data from decades and even millennia past could yield important findings and that, thus, rigorous and secondary analyses of hard-won qualitative health data is often warranted, yet rarely undertaken.

Jordan (2011) argued that examining US Civil War veterans' writings reveal "a personal effort to make sense of their injuries and the meaning behind participation in unprecedented death and dying" (126). The injuries those veterans who were fortunate enough to survive came home with were indeed unprecedented due to 19th century advances in weaponry. Explained Leonard (2012):

> Developments in arms and ammunition made battlefields far more lethal than they had been a decade before, while discoveries in medicine—which could have partially counterbalanced the awful effects of the new ordnance—were still a handful of years in the future.
>
> (n.p.)

Having suffered from exceptional injuries that led to limb loss, participants like Ritchey rightfully believed they were contributing to data that could lead to a cure for PLP. Dauntingly, though, even these many years later, much uncertainty still surrounds causes and treatments for PLP, and no treatments show entirely consistent results (Corbett et al., 2018; Kaur & Guan, 2018). Moreover, while many researchers have described, studied, and acknowledged PLP as a global phenomenon, "there is still no detailed explanation of its mechanisms" (Kaur & Guan, 2018, p. 368). That said, remarkably, the viable theories and knowledges that do exist on PLP causes and treatments today are hinted at in the survey responses many decades before they appeared in the literature.

Moreover, much like the participants in Chapter 3, the veterans whose survey responses are examined in this chapter engage in important rhetorical work when they attempt to strengthen *ethos* that had been damaged due to amputation and PLP. As Carroll (2017) explained, "Many disabled Civil War veterans felt embarrassed and shamed of their disability, and even a prosthetic limb could not fill the deep void an amputated limb could leave" (n.p.). The perplexing reality of living with debilitating PLP added to this social suffering. Just as misunderstood in the popular imagination as in the clinical literature, Graham (2015) described PLP as "cited over and over again at the beginning of academic, medical, and popular treatises devoted to describing the puzzle of pain, the mystery of pain, and the war on pain" (p. 117). Indeed, the idea that a person could feel pain in a body part that is no longer there does present a unique etiological mystery and brings up myriad questions on the relationship between psychiatric trauma and physical symptoms.

As Chapter 3 demonstrated, patients overcome assumptions of their credibility due to demographic factors beyond their control by strategically preparing for and performing in clinical appointments and by reconfiguring their *ethos* from "hysterical" patient to astute advocate. In most cases, participants in the interview study described in Chapter 3 needed to recover credibility that had been unfairly damaged by the erroneous assumption—often based on race, class, and/or gender biases—that their symptoms were "all in their heads" when, in fact, the vast majority were eventually given physical health diagnoses that accounted for their symptoms. As Chapter 2 made clear, the misdiagnosis of mental health problems in the medically ill is linked to often tacit forms of discrimination. While both Chapters 2 and 3 gesture toward the stigmatizing nature of disabilities, neither provides a clear portrait of how those with known physical disabilities contend with problematic, inaccurate ideas about their mental well-being, nor do these chapters do more than make passing mention of the complexity of diagnosis in terms of body-mind dualism. PLP presents an opportunity to meditate on such things.

Moreover, as this book seeks to showcase the versatility and utility of examining everyday appeals to *ethos* across health and medical contexts toward original theories-building, this chapter adds important temporal depth by bringing vernacular voices buried in an archive into the discussion. This chapter, thus, examines PLP by analyzing US Civil War amputees' tacit strategies for establishing *ethos* following the stigmatizing experiences of wartime limb loss. More specifically, this chapter's data is comprised of surveys US Civil War veterans, referenced above, filled out several decades post-amputation with the intention of sharing the "remote consequences" of their injuries with researchers (Mitchell,

1863–1906). I examined these documents in the papers of S. Weir Mitchell, 19th century physician and leading specialist on injuries of the nerves. These artifacts, which are housed in the Philadelphia College of Physicians archives (Mitchell, 1863–1906), like other objects of vernacular inquiry, examine "the language used to talk as opposed to the language used to talk about" (Ingraham, 2013, p. 13). As such, this chapter examines the men's own responses to PLP rather than relying on clinical observations from their doctors. The surveys, thus, provide a snapshot of amputees' particular descriptions of their physical and mental states in the years post-amputation. Importantly, these descriptions predict future clinical findings on PLP and, therefore, demonstrate the value of vernacular archival health data for illuminating contemporary clinical knowledge—particularly as the data relate to body-mind connection and complicated clinical presentation. They also make a case for the potential value of secondary analyses of qualitative health data as a way to both further clinical knowledge and to elevate and ennoble participants' contributions.

These surveys reveal astute observations on the nature of the condition of PLP and a broad range of postwar issues worth further exploration. Though they haven't been the subject of much scholarly work, a recent essay on these phantom limb surveys in the *Journal of Trauma and Dissociation* (Bonnan-White, Yep, & Hetzel-Riggin, 2016) uses these surveys to retrospectively diagnose respondents with traumatic disorders. As the authors explained, the surveys "although limited in scope . . . illustrate a history of veteran experience with physical trauma, medical treatment, coping mechanisms, posttraumatic stress, dissociation, and negotiating social stigma" (p. 25). This chapter similarly works retroactively, but the focus is on showing these men's appeals to *ethos* in ways that highlight their mental wellness and their astute self-knowledge rather than in ways that indicate contemporary mental health-related diagnostic categories. Importantly, too, a present-day read of the surveys shows that the men were able to anticipate current clinical findings on PLP such as, for example, that the phenomenon very likely has physical causes and that the pain is related to the perceived inability to move the phantom limb. Read through the lens of rhetorical *ethos*, these men's words reveal their awareness of stigma and its role in their suffering. Having this knowledge led them to embed counterarguments to that stigma in their survey responses.

Arguably, these men's experiences with stigma stem not only from their status of less-than-fully-human in the eyes of their 19th century contemporaries, but also from their claims to maintaining feeling in their missing limbs. Seeming to be aware of the fact that admitting to having pain in what they often referred to as their "missing members," these veterans were able to use the space of the surveys to make important appeals to *ethos*. In so doing, they demonstrated that their disabled subjectivities did not diminish their personhood, that their overall health remained intact following amputation, and that their status as disabled had a lot to do with the inferiority of the prosthetic technologies available to them. Prior to sharing this data, it is necessary to, first, describe its origins and its original context.

Some Background on PLP, S. Weir Mitchell, and the Surveys

Given its still-confounding status in contemporary clinical literature, it is interesting to note that PLP has been well documented for hundreds of years. While the first description of the phenomenon of experiencing pain in a missing limb is attributed to 16th century French military surgeon Ambroise Paré, it was 19th century Philadelphia physician S. Weir Mitchell, a leading 19th century specialist on injuries of the nerves—who coined the term "PLP" (Finger & Hustwit, 2003). Dauntingly, despite the intervening years of research, PLP remains in many ways as etiologically shrouded in mystery as it was in the 19th century, as the literature on PLP is inconsistent; it either attributes the phenomenon to physical causes, to psychological causes, or to both. Ishinova (2018) argued that PLP can be "caused by the emotional condition of patients and the particulars of their personality" (p. 18). Other researchers are more confident in PLP's classification as "neuropathic pain following amputation" (Osumi et al., 2018). Indeed, Kuffler (2018) explained that "various studies suggest that PLP is triggered by changes in the nervous system" (p. 67).

That said, popular representations in television would seem to suggest that the *doxa* or popular opinion surrounding PLP is that it is a purely psychological condition. The erroneous misattribution of psychological problems in amputees, of course, is likely due, in some part, to the uncharitable belief that living without a limb constitutes a significant and irreparable psychic injury and that a physically disabled person could not possibly be mentally well—a viewpoint that is hostile to disability studies' aim, as described in Chapter 1, of emphasizing that built environments and negative social dispositions toward difference are problematically disabling (Dolmage, 2009, 2015). Thus, the popular belief that limb loss renders a person irredeemably damaged in terms of mental health leads to the misconception that those with PLP are experiencing mental illness when they claim to feel pain in, say, a leg that is no longer there.

For example, in a 2013 episode of the popular American television show *Grey's Anatomy* (Rhimes & Hardy, 2013), lead character Dr. Meredith Grey opined:

> Patients who undergo amputation often feel sensation where the missing limb was, as if it's still there. The syndrome is called phantom limb. It's as if the body can't accept that a terrible trauma has occurred. The mind is trying to make the body complete again. Patients who experience phantom limb report many different sensations, but by far the most common is pain.

Clearly, this episode represents PLP as a trauma response and insinuates that the pain originates in the person's "mind." Hundreds of years before that episode aired, Mitchell (2015b) also famously wrote a fictional account of a man he called George Dedlow; as this fictional war veteran described it, "This pain keeps the brain ever mindful of the missing part, and, imperfectly at least, preserves to the man a consciousness of possessing that which he has not" (p. 139). Thus, Mitchell's fictional account, published in *Atlantic* magazine in 1866, likely perpetuated the idea that PLP is a mental health issue by implying that the phantom limb is a trick the mind is playing on the body. In both cases, the implication is that the person's mind cannot accept the now "imperfect" body and the pain isn't real, but a specter. Interestingly, though, for Mitchell, a "theory that the mind and body are one determined his clinical treatment. In Western medicine, of course, this sentiment is often absent" (Cervetti, 2003, p. 90). That said, Mitchell did not intend to publish the Dedlow story. Instead, a friend with whom Mitchell shared the story sent it to the magazine. That is, Mitchell did not intentionally contribute to the idea of PLP as a purely psychological problem, yet his story undoubtedly led to its entry into *doxa* as such—a sentiment that has proven, in contemporary shows like *Grey's Anatomy*, to have staying power.

Despite this *doxa* that suggests PLP is a purely psychological condition, and Mitchell's own hand in creating that misconception, he coined the term to refer to what he believed to be a psychiatric and physiological phenomenon wherein those who'd lost limbs still felt sensations in their missing members due to nerve pain as well as psychological distress. The word "phantom," though, was not an effective term to convey that belief as it likely contributed and continues to contribute to the idea that sensations in missing limbs are akin to hauntings and apparitions and are equally as suspect. In fact, perhaps the stigma the word "phantom" inevitably carries when it is attached to a subjective report of a bodily sensation is one of the reasons why it is sometimes called "post-amputation limb pain" in clinical literature today. Despite the pitfalls of the word "phantom," Mitchell's clinical writings reveal that he believed that nerve damage as well as what we would today call psychiatric trauma were responsible for the manifestation of phantom pains.

"In many," reflected Mitchell (2015a), "the limb may be recalled to the man by irritating the nerves in the stump" (p. 147). Thus, Mitchell clearly saw a physical relationship between the system of nerves remaining in the stump and PLP. However, he also felt that the condition was nonetheless mysterious and frightening. Recalling a man whose shoulder was given an electrical shock and who, then, felt his missing hand as if it were present and in intense pain, Mitchell (2015a) remarked, "No resurrection of the dead, no answer of a summoned spirit, could have been more startling" (p. 148). Mitchell's work introduces an important interdisciplinary point of thinking—if no medical answer is present, then is this a question that can be answered by medicine? Or is this an experience better answered by philosophy or rhetoric? Or even religion or faith? Still, Mitchell persisted in examining PLP as a medical phenomenon, providing further evidence in his belief that PLP, though confounding, had physical etiologies.

According to his biographer Cervetti (2003), Mitchell took the discomfort of his war veteran patients very seriously. Contemporary anesthesiologists, thus, consider Mitchell a "pioneer" in their expanding field of practice. Better known for his work with "hysteric" female patients in his controversial "rest cure,"[1] Mitchell thought and wrote tirelessly on injuries of the nerves and pain, coining not only the term "PLP," but "causalgia"—a term for burning pain. Still, today, even though most amputees experience PLP, the "literature reporting on PLP data is relatively spartan" (Aldington et al., 2014, p. 39). In terms of pain management for those with PLP, moreover, "treatment does not achieve the typical goals of the population" and most contemporary treatments are considered "analgesic failures" (Aldington et al., 2014, p. 41). Just as survey participants were quite optimistic about the prospects of their contributions leading to a cure, the relative lack of progress in the understanding and treatment of PLP today would undoubtedly disappoint Mitchell if he were alive. In his 1872 volume *Injuries of the Nerves and Their Consequences*, Mitchell (1872) lamented the unclear etiology of phantom limbs, noting that clinicians must "treat the pain alone, without true knowledge of its immediate causes" (p. 266). With remarkable foresight, Mitchell (2015a) explained:

> In full health we receive in the brain, when we move a part, impressions of the force exerted, the position gained, and the like, which are messages from the part moved, and which at once become of value in regulating, directing or checking the movement. The nerves which carry such information to the head sensations which, seeming to come from the muscle of the lost limb, create in the brain the illusion of their having moved.
>
> (p. 148)

A veteran who'd identified himself only with the initials HSH wrote to Mitchell to offer a description that might have led to Mitchell's thinking: "in my dreams, I remain a man with a perfect frame" (Hicks, 2011, p. 557). While he did not suffer from PLP himself, then, these and similar sentiments preoccupied Mitchell. He desperately wanted to find a clear cause and logical course of treatment for this condition. In order to learn more about this mysterious pain, Mitchell and his colleagues George Read Morehouse and William Williams Keen systematically observed the Union soldier amputees they were fortunate enough to work with at the Turner's Lane Military Hospital in Philadelphia. Explained Hicks (2011), "The first hospital to treat nerve injuries, Turner's Lane created a body of work that effectively founded American neurology" (p. 555). Although treatments for PLP developed at Turner's Lane were far from ideal, "they were usually better than the absolute neglect of such conditions, which was the standard of the day" (Schoenberg, 1997, p. 8).

In the immediate post-US Civil War period, of course, pain management was rather rudimentary—even when the physiological origins for pain were rather clear. However, as Schoenberg (1997) explained, "the rise of humanitarianism, individualism and comprehensive egalitarianism, the softening of religious predeterminism, the influence of Romanticism in the arts, and the vast sweeping social reforms associated with the maturation of the Industrial Revolution" made a focus on pain management more likely during the Civil War than it had been previously; post-Civil War, "pain no longer had the meaning it once did as a sacrifice for the common good and thus it became acceptable to seek to control it" (Schoenberg, 1997, p. 9). What remained a symbol of sacrifice to some, however, were the empty sleeves and prosthetic legs that were stark reminders of the war's various casualties. Some Union veterans saw their empty sleeves as symbolic; in a material-rhetorical sense, some veterans even used the visceral realities of their missing limbs as visual arguments to resist resolution (Jordan, 2011, p. 124). The surveys housed in Mitchell's archives offer a rare glimpse at these veterans' day-to-day experiences with PLP, with prosthetics, and with health and wellness in general, and this data shows complexity beyond the symbolic use of the missing limb in public deliberations.

Interestingly, although they have been attributed to Mitchell himself, archival material that accompanies the 1893 questionnaires that are housed in Mitchell's archives strongly suggest that they were actually collected by his son John—also a physician—as a follow-up study of amputees his father and colleagues George Read Morehouse and William Williams Keen treated at Turner's Lane to learn more about what he called the "remote consequences" of amputation (Mitchell, 1895). These surveys were collected nearly three decades after amputation, yet they bring intimate details of participants' subjective experiences with pain and post-amputation care to light. As well, they reveal how veterans understood their conditions on the organic/somatoform spectrum. In these questionnaires, thus, the younger physician is able to use his father's research as a starting point to capture discursive moments wherein veterans describe and characterize some of their most daunting experiences. Their words, read through the lens of rhetorical *ethos*, become powerful predictors of future clinical findings and strong counterarguments to the stigmas surrounding their conditions.

Methods

Graham (2015) explained the distinction between pain and injury as "an artifact of the separation between mind and body" (p. 118). Crawford (2014) thus cautioned against embracing theories of phantom limbs that sacrifice "the sensorial quality of corporeality" as "residing in the body," which can lead to an overestimation of the brain as "capable of generating, of creating, everything we feel," leaving the body out of the equation, undermining social scientists' calls to bring it back in, and leading to the neglect of "a massive body of research" that starts with the idea "that we have a body and are a body" (p. 231). The danger in this line of thinking, argued Crawford, is the decontextualization of pain and pleasure and any other bodily sensation. As she succinctly puts it, "we are not reducible to the neuron" (p. 232). This chapter similarly examines the veterans' descriptions of their experiences as discursive manifestations of bodily sensations that are etiologically complex and that resist body-mind dualism. As physical symptoms in body parts that are no longer there, PLPs present a particularly compelling site for examining the relationship between physical and mental health and the attendant separation of bodies and minds.

There is a long and rich history of archival research projects and of thoughtful interrogations of archival methods and methodologies in writing and rhetoric (Cushman, 2013; Gaillet, 2012; Glenn & Enoch, 2009). Royster's (2000) work in 19th century archives of African American essayists inspired a new wave of interest in rhetorical approaches to archival projects. Enoch (2010), for example, offered a discussion of the various approaches to archival work in the field wherein scholars complicate the notion of the archival researcher as a one-dimensional "hunter or detective" in order to allow for the possibility of more complex approaches (p. 59). In response to and in line with this critical work, rhetorical researchers are often careful to portray "the archive as a fluid and emergent network, where every text resides in a network of other topical relationships and experiences" (Graban, 2013, p. 181). Jensen's (2010) powerful investigation of Progressive Era sex education initiatives and Wells's (2010) impressive examination of the health collective responsible for *Our Bodies, Ourselves* are two strong examples of RHM scholars' critical engagements with archival material. This chapter adds to this scholarship by examining archives in a way that seeks to reanimate the original research project that led to the surveys therein. It takes the everyday experiences as they are manifest in the survey responses as part of an engaged network of doctors and patients in search of answers to a confounding medical phenomenon. Rather than read the surveys as arcane curiosities, the analysis elevates the responses to the level of contemporary qualitative health data.

Moreover, as Clary-Lemon (2014) explained, "the nature of archival research is such that there is no prefabricated series of steps or theories that will apply to gathering and making sense of archival materials in every case" (p. 389). In keeping with the logics of grounded theory and with constant comparison in particular, on which the other chapters of this book also rely, I used a material approach to archival data collection and analysis that "aimed at combining object selection with ongoing interpretation of accreted layers of understanding" such that I might create "a richer base from which to make meaning out of the histories" I read in the surveys (Clary-Lemon, 2014, p. 399).

I, thus, began developing rudimentary codes while on site, in the archives, handling the original large, blue cardstock surveys (which are in remarkably good shape) and the occasional accompanying letter. While the 14 extant surveys I examined themselves took relatively little time to read through and scan, I took time to read several other items in Mitchell's archives, including letters between the famous doctor and his son John's wife Ann K. Mitchell—a woman who'd revealed, in a letter to a third party after her father-in-law's death, that S. Weir accepted far too much "self-abdication" on the part of his son. This letter helped me to make sense of an important reality of these surveys noted above— that they've been misattributed to the senior Mitchell even though the materials in the archives make it clear that John collected them. Relatedly, John's book (Mitchell, 1895) includes this dedication: "Dedicated to S. Weir Mitchell, severest of critics and kindest of fathers, that it might please him in both characters" (p. 9).

After spending a week in the archive looking through the ephemera of Mitchell's adult life (such as short notes and invitations to and from his daughter-in-law), I took scanned copies of the 14 surveys[2] and inputted them into the survey software Qualtrics—a method I used to make coding the data in NVivo a possibility. However, I also continued to read from the original handwriting of the respondents such that the materiality of the archives would not be entirely lost during analyses.

I coded the surveys for "deep self-knowledge" and for "emphasis of overall wellness." After coding was complete, I noted that "deep self-knowledge" seemed to anticipate contemporary clinical findings on PLP. I also noted that the emphasis on overall mental and physical wellness seemed related to deep dissatisfaction with available prosthetics—another successful set of appeals to *ethos*. Importantly, these sentiments revealed that the men found the interventions and treatments—and not their own states of being—to be problematic. Below, I share select results from this data coding and attendant analyses.

Deep Self-Knowledge That Anticipates Future Clinical Findings

A complication for treating PLP-related pain is heavily related to what Graham (2015) compellingly described as the reason why today's patients' subjective reports of pain are often ignored or taken as suspect. In part, the issues with credibility in certain pain reports have to do with the lack of an organic starting point or clear etiology from which a physician might prescribe a course of treatment. Just as most amputees today experience PLP (Streit et al., 2015), all 14 US Civil War veteran respondents indicated that they'd experienced PLP, and many suggested that they suffered greatly from the phenomenon. Extraordinarily, the nomenclature contemporary sufferers of PLP use to describe their pain are identical to the ones the younger Mitchell's survey participants used, such as stabbing, shooting, and burning (Mayo Clinic Staff, 2018). This survey data also suggests that participants anticipated findings to do with PLP's relationship to intricate neural networks. They hinted at physical causes for PLP, and they also knew that the pain was related to the inability to move and manipulate the missing limb.

For example, as survey respondent ED Watkins explained, "It feels as if the foot is in the place where amputated, can feel toes seem as tied or bandaged." Henry Kircher similarly wrote of his phantom fingers, "I cannot clinch them to make a fist nor strengthen the fingers altogether. When I attempt these movements, the nerves in stump move." Richard Dunphy's phantom fingers felt "all grouped together around," and Stanford Pettibone felt like "feet were at the end of stumps, but terribly cramped."

The men, thus, seemed to know that the pain came from not being able to move the missing limb or phantom and that their mind misconstrued the reality of the amputation—lines of thinking that anticipated a focus of much contemporary research into PLP, the "neuromatrix," which is essentially the brain's map of the body that dictates its sensations.[3] In other words, as described above, the brain, say some neuroscientists, has a map of the body. When the map includes limbs that are not present, the brain (not the amorphous mind) forms sensations and pain in existing nerves in response (Wareham & Sparkes, 2018). Compellingly, this explanation is also used to explain the condition apotemnophilia—the drive to amputate a healthy limb; some researchers say that the limb fails to appear in the brain's image of the body, so the person has a compulsion to amputate (Tatu & Bogousslavsky, 2018).

Just as the men indicated that, if only they could move and manipulate the missing member, they might find relief, a contemporary treatment for PLP is mirror box therapy, which works on this same premise of the brain's distress at finding a missing body part that remains mapped internally, yet missing and contorted and/or paralyzed. In mirror box therapy, a mirror image of the remaining limb is used to convince the brain that the missing limb also remains and retains manipulability; research has suggested that it is an inexpensive, low-tech, successful model (Lamont, Chin, & Kogan, 2011).

Mirror box therapy originated in Ramachandran and Rogers-Ramachandran (1996) where the researchers found that mirror boxes, meant to allow patients to, for example, unclench a phantom hand via unclenching the intact hand (and its reflection in the mirror), brought immense relief, leading the researchers to argue that mirror box therapy's successes validated a more dynamic, interactive model where neural changes are possible (p. 386). It is important to recognize the fact that all of the technology required for mirror box therapy existed in the 19th century, when these men offered the very insights that could have led to a similar intervention.

Virtual reality rehabilitation,[4] an update on mirror therapy with enhanced features for healing, works under the auspices of the same logics—that PLP is the result of a mismatch between the body and brain and attendant never damage and should be treated accordingly. As Osumi and colleagues (2018) put it, "PLP patients experienced illusory perceptions of voluntarily moving their phantom limb" through virtual reality rehabilitation, "which led to restoration of phantom limb movement" (p. 5), though this treatment is not successful for all patients (p. 8).[5] The idea of using a mirror or virtual reality technologies to treat a "phantom" condition brings its own rhetorical and symbolic connections, of course. A mirror represents some truth or reality, yet it is simultaneously a falsehood, a chimera. It might even be read as a psychological trick rather than a remedy based in brain science. Thus, it is a particularly compelling site, within PLP, to consider body-mind dualism. Since it is purported to work on the basis of a physical brain and system of nerves receiving confirming visual information to remedy a mismatch between what is expected to be there and what is actually there, it is a treatment that rides the line between body-based and mind-based therapies.

Contemporary studies have "consistently suggested the importance of restoring voluntary movement of a phantom limb as the underlying mechanism of PLP alleviation," but the analgesic outcome of such treatments has shown inconsistent results (Osumi et al., 2018, p. 2). Still, it is remarkable that these men—responding to a mail-in survey over a hundred years ago—were able to accurately describe what is widely accepted today to be a defining clinical feature of PLP and were able to offer descriptions through which the most promising treatments of the condition might have evolved much sooner. These men's descriptions of their PLP experiences clearly indicated that the pain related to the inability to "move" the missing part. In this way, these respondents demonstrated deep bodily knowledge resembling *metis*. As de Certeau (1984) described it, metis "draws its knowledge from a multitude of events among which it moves without possessing them . . . it also computes and predicts the multiple paths of the future;" it is "an accumulation of time" and it has the capacity to "concentrate the most knowledge in the least time" (p. 83). While even today, say researchers, "little is known about the potentially unique healthcare needs" of amputees with PLP (Katon & Reiber, 2013, p. 173), knowing and trusting their bodies, these men arguably knew as much or more about PLP's mechanisms in the 1890s as researchers do today, and metis as "cunning and adaptive intelligence" (Dolmage, 2014, p. 5) helps to account for this reality. These men, then, had epistemological affordances for making sense of PLP that researchers who'd never experienced it could simply not have. These ways of knowing formed by slow accretion from the time of injury, through the years of navigating their new realities, to the time they received a survey in the mail and were able to offer up their thoughts.

Emphasizing Overall Wellness and Inconvenience of Artificial Limb Design as Disabling

Survey respondents' matter-of-fact descriptions of how they came to be amputees included various kinds of gunshot wounds and lacerations. They described feet lost to frostbite, crushing, or mashing. They wrote about arms lost to the bursting of a shell. As Willis W. Owens reported in a letter sent back to the researchers with the blank survey, he'd undergone eleven thorough interviews and examinations as part of the pension process, and his comrades likely were subjected to the same. Through repeatedly recounting their stories of injury and amputation, the men were likely practiced at using words and phrases that would signal real distress and need. Still, in the surveys, which the men knew to be for research for a cure, the men chose to emphasize their wellness. Henry Kircher, for example, is clear in his assessment of his health: "I enjoy good health cannot say that loss of limbs made any changes in health," and Clark Gardner noted "no appreciable change other than from age" and that his "sleep is natural" and his "appetite is good."

Recognizing that others perceived them as damaged in general from their limb loss, survey respondents emphasized their overall health and wellness despite amputation to establish their credibility. Likewise, they emphasized the inconvenience of the artificial limbs—a move that implied that if these prosthetics were better, they'd have better lives. These appeals to *ethos* worked to undercut stigma that followed their limb loss—stigma that would suggest that they are so damaged physically and mentally and, thus, have little remaining value. Instead, relaying how difficult available prosthetics were to live with allowed them to tacitly suggest that they'd fare better with more and better accommodations. Indeed, Carroll (2017) shared a poignant story of veteran Walter Lenoir. In 1862, Lenoir lost his leg after being hit with a Minié ball. As Carroll explained:

> Lenoir was justifiably afraid that his injury would leave him crippled, unloved, and alone. His fear was justifiable—Lenoir lived in a culture that valued the whole body as a mark of manliness. To Americans living in the late nineteenth century, disability could be a window into character. A limp or an amputation could be evidence of moral degeneration as well as physical harm.
>
> (n.p.)

In this context, the men's descriptions of their wellness in body and mind can be read as rebuffs to such stigmas. The survey asked participants, for example, "Has the loss of your member altered the general health? Have there been any alterations of pulse? body temperature? digestion? intellectual powers? disposition? or habits?" Though some noted changes, most respondents did not report alterations in general health. Frank Mark responded, "Not materially" and Lewis Atherton reported, "have never been as robust or strong." Another question asked: "Has there been any change in the acuteness of the special senses i.e. hearing, sight, sense of taste?" A related question asked: "What reason have you for ascribing such alterations, if any are noted, to the injury or operation?" Most responses to the first of these related questions are negative, as perhaps respondents wished to emphasize how much of their former selves they had retained. While six respondents noted changes in hearing, some attribute that change to injury and others simply to age. Later on, the survey asked, "Is there any alteration in the amount of sleep, or of solid or liquid nourishment required?" To this question, six responded that there had been no alteration while others note a need for more sleep.

A final, related question asked, "Was the amputation followed by any marked change in your ability for mental or bodily exertion?" One participant reported that he was "entirely disabled," another noted fatigue, a third wrote "pain at mental study," yet the majority did not attribute any changes in mental or bodily exertion to the injury. One respondent, in fact, made his response very clear: that "none except from loss of members" have been altered.

The US federal government offered artificial limbs to all Union amputees;[6] these were given in the hopes of making amputees feel whole again. Prosthetics were to help the men function better, but they also were meant to help the men to blend in socially (Figg & Farrell-Beck, 1993). However, as Kircher made clear, nothing will replace that which has been lost, and that must be acknowledged. With pragmatism and a hint of sarcasm, when asked which artificial appendage was most satisfactory, Kircher responded "My old bone and flesh leg." Richard Dunphy tentatively appreciated his prosthetics. He recalled them as painful and inconvenient, but he noted that, with their use, he "could do [his] own writing and feed [him]self." However, the vast majority of respondents found their prosthetics to be a problem. Lewis Atherton found his to be "tiresome, of no use." Elsewhere, the missing limbs were symbolic of the men's service and sacrifice, but they indicated that they felt rather left behind and really wanted to know what was causing such great suffering; they felt that there must be a viable physical treatment. Henry Kircher replied to a question on pain following injury, "of course it hurt"—a response that indicates that, though he's been through a painful experience—one that would be painful to anyone—he remained a rational and clear-minded individual. In short, they came across, in my reading, as decidedly resisting what we'd today call "traumatized subjectivities."

"In contrast to the many works that psychiatrists and historians, philosophers and anthropologists have devoted to the subject" of trauma,

Fassin and Rechtman (2009) explained that "the truth of trauma lies not in the psyche, the mind, or the brain, but in the moral economy of contemporary societies" (p. 275). That is, trauma draws all of its energy from its interpretation. Emphasizing their wellness of body and mind, these men perhaps wished to show that they'd successfully survived what we'd call incredibly traumatic experiences, yet wanted to express that they did not feel irrevocably affected. These men had clear dissatisfaction with the lethargy and inertia of their lives post-war, and much of that seemed to stem not from their health, which most said was fine other than the missing limb, but to the poor design of prosthetics available at the time.

Conclusion

Lamenting the fact that despite a healthy amount of interdisciplinary health research on PLP, relatively little is systematically known or accepted as scientific fact, Kaur and Guan (2018) presented a systematic review to synthesize existing knowledge. Their conclusions fit with other assertions of the phenomenon's organic etiologies and, thus, the survey respondents' beliefs in organic causes for their phantom pains: "It is unsurprising that with an amputation that such an intricate highway of information transport to and from the periphery may have potential for problematic neurologic developments," and while "no concise conclusion" yet exists on PLP, researchers have pointed to various potential causes in the sympathetic nervous system (p. 2).

Noting that "phantom limbs are enigmatic and intriguing, for they depict missing body parts whose existence is subserved by illusory sensory perceptions for which objective evidence is necessarily unattainable," (p. 960), Schott (2014) explored how images those who've experienced PLP create of their phantom limbs "validate what are otherwise solely patients' anecdotal accounts, whether verbal or written" (p. 961). Metaphor, such as a drawing of a toe being smashed with a hammer, has been used to attempt to make PLP suffering more intelligible (p. 966). There was likely similar clinical value in the survey respondents' descriptions of their PLP, such as in Chat Ritchey's creative and enigmatic explanation of his PLP as "double geared lightning."

Still, in examining the sensory experiences of the Civil War, historian Smith (2014) cautioned that "the meaning people attached to certain sensory experiences in, say, 1863 cannot be understood with the same or even similar meaning today" (p. 3). Nonetheless, Bonnan-White and colleagues (2016) urged others to take these surveys seriously, asking "traumatologists and related practitioners to take a moment to hear these voices amplified only by fountain pen scratched on 150-year-old paper" (p. 30). While I agree with Bonnan-White and colleagues' assessment, this chapter uses rhetorical lenses alongside the surveys to further examine the contribution these surveys made and to theorize the contributions they might have made beyond indicating psychiatric problems in the respondents.

Moreover, while there is merit in working to establish and legitimize the psychic suffering of US Civil War veterans by retroactively assigning them a contemporary clinical mental health diagnosis, this chapter has been more interested in how their astute observations of their bodily experiences anticipate future clinical findings on PLP, namely that the phenomenon likely has physical causes due to nerve damage and that pain was related to not being able to perceive movement in the missing limb. The data, thus, suggests that perhaps there is important knowledge to be gained from examining these surveys and other archival health data via the lens of rhetorical *ethos*. As this inquiry examines qualitative health research conducted in the 19th century, the data also reveals the inadequate reciprocity of this kind of research. The data shows, that is, that the participants expected to see the results of the research to which they generously contributed offer them relief in their lifetimes. Sharing their everyday bodily experiences can be read (as I've read it) as remarkably prescient since it seems to predict clinical findings that were many decades away. Still, another way to interpret the realties that these vernacular contributions to research convey is that too often, the data we collect is more valuable than most analyses can reveal. The lessons learned from this archival research might, thus, be to spend more time analyzing and parsing data from similar projects. Doing so could be an effort to ensure that contemporary researchers do not miss an important finding that is embedded in a person's everyday experiences of a health and medical phenomenon. Indeed, in opposition to the vernacular, which he defined as "language that talks," Ingraham (2013) described the way that:

> The elite wields the power in part because theirs is the language that talks about, and such specialized language is the language that confers status, which is then distinguished, in an ongoing cycle, by the language it uses to understand itself and validate (value) the social conversation around it.
>
> (p. 6)

A similar dynamic exists between the researcher and the researched, and care must be taken to elevate contributions to qualitative health research such that it is taken as potentially powerful in terms of its capacity to revolutionize clinical thinking on mystifying conditions. In some ways, the US Civil War PLP artifacts make it clear that, in health and medicine, there can be the illusion that research can and should yield answers long before it actually does. With that being the case, health research participants might even agree to participate due to the too-often erroneous assumption that they themselves and their contemporaries will benefit from the research. Again, considered today to be an "analgesic failure" (Aldington et al., 2014, p. 41), PLP is still relatedly misunderstood—particularly in *doxa* or popular opinion—as a mental health issue that has its origins in the trauma event (illness or injury) that led to the amputation to begin with, rather than as a physical issue. These men's everyday descriptions of their experiences with PLP counter these misunderstandings.

These survey respondents, then, were supplying answers based on their everyday experiences to the researchers they hoped would provide some relief from their often daunting and debilitating suffering. The PLP these veterans experienced would seem to point to feelings of extreme frustration with the inertia that war experience and amputation inflicted on their lives. Emphasizing their overall wellness and problems with inadequate prosthetics, they show that the issues that accompany their status as amputees exceed them and that if interventions were improved, their lives could be better. These archival materials further suggest that today's veterans' vernacular descriptions of their combat-related injuries of the body and mind very likely deserve more focused attention.

Like US Civil War amputees, contemporary veterans worldwide with marks of difference, such as physical or mental disability, are unfairly stigmatized and, thus, considered unreliable. Operation Enduring Freedom and Operation Iraqi Freedom (OEF/OIF) combat veterans who've sought treatment for post-traumatic stress disorder (PTSD) report that stigma and stereotypes of their conditions that suggest they are dangerous, violent, or crazy can be so strong as to deter help-seeking behavior (Mittal et al., 2013).

As well, while some contemporary amputees take full advantage of advancements in prosthetics to elevate their standing to adaptive athletes or even superathletes—to not only regain their lost functionality, but to surpass it—others suffer from issues with psychosocial adjustment. Indeed, researchers have found that mental health concerns can arise post-amputation due to perceived social stigma and body image issues (Rybarczyk, Nyenhuis, Nicholas, Cash, & Kaiser, 1995, p. 107). Galli, Reel, Henderson, and Detling's (2016) interview study showed that while athletic involvement can help amputees and other disabled persons improve feelings of self-worth, there are still significant body image issues in amputees due, in large part, to social standards. As they explained:

> Able-bodied individuals or those with milder disabilities had stronger body esteem than individuals with more severe disabilities. These findings suggest that as individuals' bodies stray further from stereotypical notions of the able-bodied norm, they experience more negative feelings about their bodies. Limb amputation may also be associated with negative body image, as amputees may feel that their bodies no longer align with societal conceptions of a healthy body.
>
> (Galli et al., 2016, p. 2)

These archival materials might help to argue for the value of learning directly from the everyday experiences of today's global war veterans. If such studies are undertaken, this data suggests that future clinical findings on combat-related suffering of body and mind might even be embedded in present everyday descriptions of veterans' experiences. Likewise, valuable strategies for rebuilding credibility after traumatic war experiences are likely discernable in contemporary veterans' everyday talk.

Notes

1. The "rest cure," in fact, was made especially famous when 19th century feminist author Charlotte Perkins Gilman composed the story "The Yellow Wallpaper" based on her experiences in Mitchell's care.
2. It is important to address the limited size of this data set. That said, its rarity makes it nonetheless worthy of study.
3. Congenital amputees complicate this portrait since plasticity would indicate that the neuromatrix would not include the limbs for which some still feel phantoms.
4. Another contemporary finding led to targeted reinnervation—a treatment for difficulty with prosthetic limb function. This treatment follows the logics of PLP as an organic phenomenon related to intricate neural networks. The survey respondents' visceral knowledge of PLP led them to describe the relationship between PLP and the nerves in the stump. As a "neural-machine interface," targeted reinnervation "rewires peripheral nerves and uses available surface muscles as biological amplifiers to develop rich new sources of motor command signals" (Kuiken et al., 2007, p. 378). After receiving this therapy, explained Kuiken et al. (2007), the participant in their case study "found that her prosthetic was much easier and more natural to use, because she was using physiologically appropriate neural pathways to operate her artificial limb" (p. 378).
5. Importantly, while mirror therapy is simple, affordable and effective, the clinical data is not as strong as researchers would like (Campo-Prieto & Rodriguez-Fuentes, 2018).
6. Confederate amputees relied on state support for prosthetics for many years.

References

Aldington, D., Small, C., Edwards, D., Ralph, J., Woods, P., Jagdish, S., Moore, R. A. (2014). A survey of post-amputation pains in serving military personnel. *Journal of the Royal Army Medical Corps*, 160(1), 38–41. doi:10.1136/jramc-2013-000069

Bonnan-White, J., Yep, J., & Hetzel-Riggin, M. D. (2016). Voices from the past: Mental and physical outcomes described by American Civil War amputees. *Journal of Trauma & Dissociation*, 17(1), 13–34. doi:10.1080/1529973 2.2015.1041070.

Campo-Prieto, P., & Rodriguez-Fuentes, G. (2018). Effectiveness of mirror therapy in phantom limb pain: A literature review. *Neurologia* (Epub ahead of print), doi: S0213-4853(18)30201–9 [pii]

Carroll, D. (2017, February 23). After the amputation. Retrieved from www.civilwarmed.org/prosthetics/

de Certeau, M. (1984). *The practice of everyday life*. Berkeley: University of California Press.

Cervetti, N. (2003). S. Weir Mitchell representing "a hell of pain": From civil war to rest cure. *Arizona Quarterly: A Journal of American Literature, Culture, and Theory, 59*(3), 69–96. doi:10.1353/arq.2003.0001.

Clary-Lemon, J. (2014). Archival research processes: A case for material methods. *Rhetoric Review, 33*(4), 381–402. doi:10.1080/07350198.2014.946871.

Collins, K. L., Russell, H. G., Schumacher, P. J., Robinson-Freeman, K. E., O'Conor, E. C., Gibney, K. D., . . . Tsao, J. W. (2018). A review of current theories and treatments for phantom limb pain. *The Journal of Clinical Investigation, 128*(6), 2168–2176. doi:10.1172/JCI94003.

Corbett, M., South, E., Harden, M., Eldabe, S., Pereira, E., Sedki, I., . . . Woolacott, N. (2018). Brain and spinal stimulation therapies for phantom limb pain: A systematic review. *Health Technology Assessment, 22*(62), 1–94. doi:10.3310/hta22620.

Crawford, C. (2014). *Phantom limb: Amputation, embodiment, and prosthetic technology*. New York: New York University Press.

Cushman, E. (2013). Wampum, Sequoyan, and story: Decolonizing the digital archive. *College English, 76*(2), 115–135. Retrieved from www.jstor.org/stable/24238145

Dolmage, J. (2009). Metis, mêtis, mestiza, medusa: Rhetorical bodies across rhetorical traditions. *Rhetoric Review, 28*(1), 1–28. doi:10.1080/07350190802540690.

Dolmage, J. (2014). *Disability rhetoric*. Syracuse, NY: Syracuse University Press.

Dolmage, J. (2015). Universal design: Places to start. *Disability Studies Quarterly, 35*(2). doi:10.18061/dsq.v35i2.4632.

Enoch, J. (2010). Changing research methods, changing history: A reflection on language, location, and archive. *Composition Studies, 38*(2), 47–73. Retrieved from www.jstor.org/stable/compstud.38.2.0047

Fassin, D., & Rechtman, R. (2009). *The empire of trauma*. Princeton, NJ: Princeton University Press.

Figg, L., & Farrell-Beck, J. (1993). Amputation in the civil war: Physical and social dimensions. *Journal of the History of Medicine and Allied Sciences, 48*(4), 454–475. doi:10.1093/jhmas/48.4.454.

Finger, S., & Hustwit, M. P. (2003). Five early accounts of phantom limb in context: Paré, Descartes, Lemos, Bell, and Mitchell. *Neurosurgery, 52*(3), 686. doi:10.1227/01.neu.0000048478.42020.97.

Gaillet, L. L. (2012). (Per)forming archival research methodologies. *College Composition and Communication, 64*(1), 35–58. Retrieved from www.jstor.org/stable/23264916

Galli, N., Reel, J. J., Henderson, H., & Detling, N. (2016). An investigation of body image in athletes with physical disabilities. *Journal of Clinical Sport Psychology, 10*(1), 1–18. doi:10.1123/JCSP.2015-0018.

Glenn, C., & Enoch, J. (2009). Drama in the archives: Rereading methods, rewriting history. *College Composition and Communication, 61*(2), 321–342. Retrieved from www.jstor.org/stable/40593445

Graban, T. S. (2013). From location(s) to loanability: Mapping feminist recovery and archival activity through metadata. *College English, 76*(2), 171–193. Retrieved from www.jstor.org/stable/24238148

Graham, S. S. (2015). *The politics of pain medicine: A rhetorical-ontological inquiry.* Chicago, IL: University of Chicago Press.

Hicks, R. D. (2011). In their dreams: The S. Weir Mitchell papers. *The Pennsylvania Magazine of History and Biography, 135*(4), 555–557. doi:10.5215/pennmaghistbio.135.4.0555.

Ingraham, C. (2013). Talking (about) the elite and mass: Vernacular rhetoric and discursive status. *Philosophy & Rhetoric, 46*(1), 1–21. doi:10.5325/philrhet.46.1.0001.

Ishinova, V. (2018). Empathy-technique: Similarity and differences of phantom limb pain and psychogenic pain. *Psychopathology and Addiction Medicine, 1*(3), 18–23. doi:10.1155/2011/864605.

Jensen, R. E. (2010). *Dirty words the rhetoric of public sex education, 1870–1924.* Urbana, IL: University of Illinois Press.

Jordan, B. M. (2011). "Living monuments": Union veteran amputees and the embodied memory of the civil war. *Civil War History, 57*(2), 121–152. doi:10.1353/cwh.2011.0025.

Katon, J. G., & Reiber, G. E. (2013). Major traumatic limb loss among women veterans and servicemembers. *Journal of Rehabilitation Research and Development, 50*(2), 173–182. doi:10.1682/JRRD.2012.01.0007.

Kaur, A., & Guan, Y. (2018). Phantom limb pain: A literature review. *Chinese Journal of Traumatology, 21*(6), 366–368. doi: S1008-1275(18)30025-7.

Kim, S. Y., & Kim, Y. Y. (2012). Mirror therapy for phantom limb pain. *The Korean Journal of Pain, 25*(4), 272–274. doi:10.3344/kjp.2012.25.4.272.

Kuffler, D. P. (2018). Origins of phantom limb pain. *Molecular Neurobiology, 55*(1), 60–69. doi:10.1007/s12035-017-0717-x.

Kuiken, T. A., Miller, L. A., Lipchitz, R. D., Lock, B. A., Stubblefield, K., Marasco, P. D., . . . Rumanian, G. A. (2007). Targeted reinnervation for enhanced prosthetic arm function in a woman with a proximal amputation: A case study. Lancet, 369(9559), 371–380. https://doi.org/10.1016/S0140-6736(07)60193-7

Lamont, K., Chin, M., & Kogan, M. (2011). Mirror box therapy: Seeing is believing. *Explore (New York, N.Y.), 7*(6), 369–372. doi:10.1016/j.explore.2011.08.002.

Leonard, P. (2012, August 31). The bullet that changed history. *New York Times.* Retrieved from https://opinionator.blogs.nytimes.com/2012/08/31/the-bullet-that-changed-history/

Mayo Clinic Staff. (2018). Phantom pain—symptoms and causes. Retrieved from www.mayoclinic.org/diseases-conditions/phantom-pain/symptoms-causes/syc-20376272

Mitchell, J. K. (1895). *Remote consequences of injuries of nerves and their treatment.* Philadelphia, PA: Lea Brothers.

Mitchell, S. W. (1863–1906). Correspondence: Series 4.5. Follow-up studies of patients with nerve injuries, 1863–1906 (Silas Weir Mitchell papers MSS 2/0241-03).

Mitchell, S. W. (1872). *Injuries of nerves and their consequences.* Philadelphia, PA: J.B. Lippincott.

Mitchell, S. W. (2015a). 'Phantom limbs'. In D. Seed, S. C. Kenny, & C. Williams (Eds.), *Life and limb* (pp. 147–148). Liverpool University Press. Retrieved from www.jstor.org/stable/j.ctt1ps3216.37

Mitchell, S. W. (2015b). The case of George Dedlow. In D. Seed, S. C. Kenny, & C. Williams (Eds.), *Life and limb* (pp. 131–146). Liverpool University Press. Retrieved from www.jstor.org/stable/j.ctt1ps3216.36

Mittal, D., Drummond, K. L., Blevins, D., Curran, G., Corrigan, P., & Sullivan, G. (2013). Stigma associated with PTSD: Perceptions of treatment seeking combat veterans. *Psychiatric Rehabilitation Journal, 36*(2), 86–92. doi:10.1037/h0094976.

Osumi, M., Inomata, K., Inoue, Y., Take, Y., Morioka, S., & Sometani, M. (2018). Characteristics of phantom limb pain alleviated with virtual reality rehabilitation. *Pain Medicine (Malden, MA)*. doi:10.1093/pm/pny269.

Ramachandran, V. S., & Rogers-Ramachandran, D. (1996). Synesthesia in phantom limbs induced with mirrors. *Royal Society, 263*(1369), 377–386.

Rhimes, S. (Producer), & Hardy, R. (Director). (2013). Walking on a dream, season 9, episode 12, Gray's Anatomy. [Video/DVD] Los Angeles, CA: Shondaland.

Royster, J. J. (2000). *Traces of a stream: Literacy and social change among African American women* (1st ed.). Pittsburgh, PA: University of Pittsburgh Press.

Rybarczyk, B., Nyenhuis, D. L., Nicholas, J. J., Cash, S. M., & Kaiser, J. (1995). Body image, perceived social stigma, and the prediction of psychosocial adjustment to leg amputation. *Rehabilitation Psychology, 40*(2), 95–110. doi:10.1037/0090-5550.40.2.95.

Schoenberg, E. (1997). The birth of scientific pain control: S. Weir Mitchell and the Turner's lane military hospital. *Bulletin of Anesthesia History, 15*(1), 8–10. doi:10.1016/S1522-8649(97)50004-7.

Schott, G. D. (2014). Revealing the invisible: The paradox of picturing a phantom limb. *Brain, 137*(3), 960–969. doi:10.1093/brain/awt244.

Smith, M. M. (2014). *The smell of battle, the taste of siege: A sensory history of the civil war.* Oxford, New York: Oxford University Press.

Streit, F., Bekrater-Bodmann, R., Diers, M., Reinhard, I., Frank, J., Wüst, S., . . . Rietschel, M. (2015). Concordance of phantom and residual limb pain phenotypes in double amputees: Evidence for the contribution of distinct and common individual factors. *The journal of pain: Official journal of the American Pain Society, 16*(12):1377–1385. http://doi.org/10.1016/j.jpain.2015.08.013

Tatu, L., & Bogousslavsky, J. (2018). Phantom sensations, supernumerary phantom limbs and apotemnophilia: Three body representation disorders. *Neurologic-Psychiatric Syndromes in Focus—Part I, 41*, 14–22. doi:10.1159/000475684.

van der Schans, C. P., Geertzen, J. H. B., Schoppen, T., & Dijkstra, P. U. (2002). Phantom pain and health-related quality of life in lower limb amputees. *Journal of Pain and Symptom Management, 24*(4), 429–436. doi://doi.org/10.1016/S0885-3924(02)00511-0.

Wareham, A. P., & Sparkes, V. (2018). Effect of one session of mirror therapy on phantom limb pain and recognition of limb laterality in military traumatic lower limb amputees: A pilot study. *Journal of the Royal Army Medical Corps.* doi:10.1136/jramc-2018-001001 [pii].

Wells, S. (2010). *Our bodies, ourselves and the work of writing* Palo Alto: Stanford University Press.

5 Recuperative *Ethos* and Agile Epistemologies in Mental Health and Beyond

Toward a Vernacular Engagement in Mental Health Ontologies[1]

Mental Illness, Stigma, and Rhetorical *Ethos*

As Chapter 1 demonstrated, rhetoricians have convincingly addressed the problems with credibility that emerge from mental illness stigma. Demonstrating that this stigma can do far more than impair *ethos*, Johnson (2010) revealed how mental illness marks a speaker with "*kakoethos*" or "anti-*ethos*" (p. 463). As she put it, stigma renders one "bad" in a "frustratingly general" sort of way; one is "worthless, evil, dirty, ugly, weak, cowardly, envious, dangerous," or other "variants of *kakos* in Greek" (p. 465). Of course, "consequences such as shame, humiliation, and decreased self-worth" are likely when stigma is present, but this outcome need not be "universal or impossible to overcome," as "much remains to be learned about the processes that fuel positive coping rather than despair on the part of those with mental illness" (Hinshaw, 2007, p. 156). This chapter examines everyday coping in the form of appeals to *ethos* in the wake of stigmatizing mental illness experiences; I call this process "recuperative *ethos*."

Reynolds (2018) pointed out that "every day something attention-getting appears to pop up about mental health in the popular press" (p. 14), making the exigence for this area of inquiry quite clear. This chapter seeks to contribute specifically to scholarship in MHRR, which, as Chapter 1 makes clear, concerns itself with vernacular ontologies and everyday rhetorics; the literature suggests that those with diagnoses ought to have agency in the discursive construction of their illnesses and lived experiences, including their courses of treatment (Prendergast, 2001; Price, 2011). This study elevates the everyday rhetorical practices of adults with chronic mental illness diagnoses and builds new theories from that ephemera.

As Pescosolido and colleagues (2010) explained, diverse constituencies working to end stigma in recent decades have operated under "the assumption that neuroscience offers the most effective tool to reduce prejudice and discrimination" (p, 1322).[2] If the general public can become convinced that mental illnesses have physiological causes, then stigma will decrease. Dauntingly, though, Pescosolido and colleagues' (2010) vignette survey research demonstrated that even though more people today equate mental illnesses with neurobiological causes, this knowledge does not change the general public's unwillingness to accept persons with mental illness diagnoses as valuable community members, viable citizens, or even worthwhile people. As Chapter 1 explained, many of Pescosolido's participants indicated, in fact, that they did not want to be in community with the mentally ill: they do not want to work with them, live near them, be friends with them, or have them marry into their families.

More recently, Pescosolido (2013) criticized the narrow focus on community and clinical interventions for ending stigma and has posited that "stigma emanates from social relationships," so "the solution to understanding and changing must similarly be embedded in changing social relationships and the structures that shape them" (15). As Mol (2002) pointed out, rhetoricians are uniquely positioned to perform original, field-based research projects that could lead to dynamic accounts of patient care; rhetorical *ethos* is one perspective through which such dynamic social relationships might be unpacked. Indeed, rhetoricians build important new theories by entering "a naturalistic field in which rhetoric occurs in order to observe, participate with, document, and analyze that rhetoric in its embodied and emplaced instantiation" (Middleton, Hess, Endres, & Senda-Cook, 2015, p. xv). This chapter examines efforts to deploy rhetorical *ethos* in day-to-day life to address the complex processes through which those with mental illnesses lose and must ultimately recover credibility in the wake of stigmatizing illness experiences.

In some ways, a discussion of *ethos*, mental illness, and recuperation resembles models of patient care that include a focus on the retrieval of the self, after mental illness experiences, but these models often rely on patient self-narration (Barker, 2003; Fardella, 2008). Similarly, studies of self-stigma and its harmful repercussions focus on the potential efficacy of expertly devised interventions and not on what might be learned from the everyday lives of those living with mental illnesses (Mittal et al., 2012; Negrini et al., 2014; Rusch et al., 2014).[3] I define recuperative *ethos*, instead, as the day-to-day discursive practices through which a person might regain credibility and, as a consequence, rebuild the personal, social, and professional standing that is often compromised in acute phases of mental illness experiences. Much like the appeals to *ethos* explored in Chapter 3, appeals to recuperative *ethos* emerge in everyday exchanges. Here, though, data unfolds in real time rather than in interviews.

Naturally, the idea that there is a stable self to lose in the first place can be read as positivist, anti-poststructuralist, and anti-postmodernity.[4] Concerns for unsound theorizing on mental health have led to scholarship that focuses on how various documents—DSM, patient records, intake forms, and the like—fail to adequately address the deceptive nature of social creations discursively constructed as immutable truths (Berkenkotter, 2008; Britzman & Pitt, 2004; Emmons, 2008; Hill, 2004; McCarthy & Gerring, 1994; Reynolds & Mari, 1989; Thompson, 2004). Likewise, rhetoricians have rightly been concerned about the unchecked proliferation of illnesses in diagnostic materials such as the DSM and the resultant hyper-medicalization of mental healthcare rhetorics (Reynolds, 2008; Berkenkotter, 2008; Segal, 2005). Overdiagnosis, of course, relies on labeling everyday behaviors pathological and on the language and rhetoric of esoteric medical expertise eclipsing the voices and experiences of persons with mental illness diagnoses. Kleinman (1988) identified this issue in his well-known distinction between "disease," which is concerned with organic origins of pathologies as they are described in medical texts, and "illness," which involves the everyday problems with living that patients encounter. The difference between these terms is an important one, as it hinges on the dissonance between people's dynamic experiences with illness and the static, organically verifiable criteria for diagnosis with a particular disease (Cassell, 1986). Like Kleinman (1988), Price (2011) relied on the complexity of lived experiences with mental illness to make convincing arguments for celebrating the neurodiversity that is left out of normative constructions of truth on mental illness and wellness. In fact, many disability studies scholars have contributed meaningful new knowledge to discussions of mental health and rhetoric; their studies also focus on elevating patients' everyday experiences as valid forms of evidence (see, for example, Holladay, 2017; Yergeau, 2017).

The study reported on in this chapter contributes to this scholarship by explicitly focusing on what Hauser (2011) called the "everyday vernacular performances" found in clinical settings. As Chapter 1 noted, Hauser promoted scholarship that examines the "texture and promise of vernacular rhetoric" (p. 159). Such scholarship, he explained, "will be concerned with the language, logic of arguments, logics of circulation, modes of evidence, modes of propriety, and stylistic devices that define issues and construct rhetorically salient meaning" (Hauser, 2011, p. 169). Employing Hauser's notion of the vernacular illuminates what Mol called "ontologies" in the unfolding of lived experiences with illnesses. For Mol, illnesses are not static; they must be traced in dynamic forms of being. As she explained, "ontology is not given in the order of things . . . ontologies are brought into being, sustained, or allowed to wither away in common, day-to-day sociomaterial practices" (2002, p. 7). The vernacular utterances I capture in the study described here, then, demonstrate Hauser's (2011) notion of vernacular rhetorics as valuable sources of meaning and Mol's idea that, for analyses that rely on ontological politics, "reality is done" via the "pivotal term . . . performance" (1998, p. 75).

Illuminating the problem of damaged *ethos* entails disentangling and tentatively sorting everyday ontologies inherent in vernacular performances of mental illnesses in ways that are responsive to Kleinman's definition of "illness." From this perspective, this chapter seeks to capture ontologies that are thinly represented or absent in written documents and published work and to track some of the performances through which rhetors re-substantiate their places in the world. These performances generate theoretical insights into the way *ethos* is established after it has been damaged and how affordances of neurodiversity play out, and these insights could be useful for diverse scholars interested in MHRR, RHM, and for various professionals working with and for vulnerable persons.

Site Description, Methods, Limitations

Like other studies of the vernacular, this field-based study seeks to elevate "everyday speech, conversations in homes, restaurants, and 'on the corner'" (Ono & Sloop, 1995, p. 20). For those with chronic mental illnesses, everyday conversations might happen in community-based, outpatient care settings. The study I describe in this chapter took place at a clubhouse. Clubhouses are outpatient community care facilities for individuals with chronic mental illnesses. They started in New York City in 1948 with the well-known Fountain House. Today, there are thousands of operational clubhouses worldwide. Most regularly recruit new members from state-run psychiatric hospitals and homeless shelters. As Popham (2014) explained, MHRR fieldwork can involve "sites of work that are fluid, ever changing, multiplicitous, oscillating" that are, thus, "difficult to categorize and circumscribe according to the static sites we might find most familiar" (2014, p. 342). In the same way, the clubhouse is a liminal space that straddles mental healthcare institution and community organization. Methodologically, I conducted a hybrid field-based study that employed naturalistic methods borrowed from anthropology as well as ethnographic methods that are much more prevalent in field-based projects in rhetoric. Thus, this chapter contributes to this book's goal of bringing together a diversity of data gathered through a variety of research methods—all in the service of showcasing the versatility and generative utility of rhetorical *ethos* as a terministic screen through which rich data gives way to new theories.

As Endres and colleagues (2016) explained:

> Since as early as the 1980s, rhetoricians have theorized the diverse, intersectional, and multimodal qualities of contemporary rhetoric by documenting, observing, participating in, and analyzing forms of in situ rhetoric.
>
> (p. 511)

Thus, rhetoricians have been doing fieldwork for quite some time. Still, field sites with vulnerable populations are uncommon and require additional ethical safeguards. This project's focus on vulnerable human subjects was met with some understandable reservations from the site director and the institutional review board (IRB).[5] To address their reservations, I designed the study in a way that allowed me to observe at the clubhouse, but not participate in clubhouse life without explicit invitation to do so from participants. I attempted to interact with participants only when they initiated conversations. I chose to draw, in this way, on naturalistic inquiry since these studies involve the "observation of people and events" in "the settings in which they would naturally occur, and involve those people who would naturally take part in them"; the goal of such studies is to capture "everyday experience" and to "detect patterns, concepts, trends, or categories that are taken as meaningful" by participants "in the course of that everyday experience" (Angrosino, 2007, p. 3).[6]

As I explain above, I blend Mol's theory of multiple ontologies (2002) with Hauser's (2011) notion of "vernacular" in order to reconstruct how those labelled mentally ill recover credibility. Generating this account meant that I "investigated my 'site' as an ethnographer, attending meetings . . . consultations, and other kinds of work"; I talked with patients and with "practitioners of various kinds" since my "aim was not to map as many details as possible, but to begin to unravel patterns in the coexistence of a variety of" mental illness experiences (Mol, 1998, p. 145).

Recognizing that rhetorical fieldwork means "engaging with the field to examine the everyday rhetorical practices that occur there" (Endres, Hess, Senda-Cook, & Middleton, 2016, p. 515), I took part in the clubhouse's day-to-day activities. The clubhouse is a rather active place. Members have "home" units where they spend much of their day, and each unit has at least one clinical staff member; these units include: business and employment, education, hospitality, and housing/homeless. Members, who far outnumber clinical staff, are free to move around the clubhouse at will, but they have responsibilities in their "home" units. These responsibilities still leave considerable free time for breaks, meals, and conversations, and much of my data was collected (with permission) during these activities. In many ways, the clubhouse made a fitting site choice for observing day-to-day interactions among adults who have mental illness diagnoses. Since many join clubhouses via local mental hospitals and homeless shelters, it constitutes a type of liminal space meant to prepare vulnerable people for life out in the community. Through opportunities for social interaction in the context of a flexible, yet meaningfully structured day, it is an ideal place to examine appeals to *ethos*. Indeed, most of the data I collected took the form of conversations among members as they navigated everyday, largely social interactions. At the clubhouse, moreover, the affordances of neurodiversity came through in ways that perhaps they would not have in more vertically arranged groups or in more traditionally clinical settings.

Each morning at the clubhouse begins with a community meeting in which all members gather in the hospitality unit—a big, open room that resembles a cafeteria. I collected data from my participants during these larger meetings. Afterward, units split off into their various places within the clubhouse building and unit members discuss the delegation of duties for the day. I spent the majority of my time in the hospitality unit where food is prepared and consumed, cleaning duties are assigned and performed, and community meetings are held. The staff member in charge of hospitality was amenable to my presence, and the clubhouse director also felt that I would have exposure to the most potential participants in this unit as all members pass through it at some point during their day. In fact, the hospitality unit backs up to the smoking gazebo, and some of my observations were made there. Thus, some of my participants were part of this unit and others came in and out for meals, meetings, and breaks.

Since attendance at the clubhouse is purely voluntary, not all members are there every day. The day itself is designed to be "work ordered" so that members can gain practice being on a schedule—something they might have lost touch with during extended hospitalizations for their chronic conditions—but that schedule is very flexible. Initially, I had planned to frame out segments of the work-ordered day—say, the lunch hour or the morning meeting—to audio-record, and these recordings were to supplement field notes. However, I was not permitted, of course, to record individuals who had not agreed to participate in my study, nor could I record those who had agreed to participate in my study, but indicated that they would be "very uncomfortable" with being recorded. As well, some members of the clubhouse ardently believed, despite my best efforts to convince them of the contrary, that I was a new member undergoing orientation and that I must have recently gotten out of the local mental hospital. In other words, they perceived my claims of being a researcher as a sign of delusion. Although some of these persons indicated an interest in participating in the study, I could not responsibly or ethically have let them do so. In my approved IRB application, I had indicated that I would be willing to "confer with clinical staff" if I was concerned about a participant's ability to offer informed consent on her or his own behalf, and I did just that. Moreover, I followed participant recruitment protocol when I believed a potential participant could be harmed through the observation. Inevitably, though, I was privy to these persons' everyday language use, and it was quite rich. I was, therefore, sorry to exclude it from the data. Ultimately, I recruited 19 participants ranging in age from 18 to 65 during the month of September 2010. These participants had diagnoses of schizophrenia, bipolar disorder, and schizoaffective disorder. This sample also included individuals from various ethnic, economic, and educational backgrounds—a sample commensurate with this clubhouse's membership in general.

In the end, I collected audio-recordings of individuals and pairs when there were one or more participants willing to be recorded and when no one present had objections to being recorded. I was often a part of the conversations that made up the audio-recordings, which likely led some participants to discuss their various roles in the community and their dispositions toward stigma. Although these recordings did not necessarily turn into interviews, they were only created when one or more participants happened to be in a room with me and no one else. In this way, they lacked some of the potency of other interactions I had the privilege of witnessing. I had to attempt, consequently, to capture significant participant interchanges in profuse field notes where I recorded as many verbatim speech acts and accurate accounts of related gestures as possible. I created these copious field notes from participants' morning routines, morning meetings, meal time, break time, smoke breaks, and work in the hospitality unit. Members invited me to participate in the hospitality unit work, so I recorded some field notes while serving food, working at the snack bar, and cleaning alongside members as well. All told, I was able to perform 180 hours of observation at the clubhouse, which led to 37 single-spaced pages of typed field notes and 99 pages of transcriptions from audio-recordings. These data capture "the micro-practices of moment-by-moment interactions" and thus "contribute not only to the organic character of the culture but become a significant source of rhetorically salient meaning and influence" (Hauser, 2011, p. 159).

What these documents do not capture are the memories I have of those hours of observation. Many participants had materially and economically challenging lives; they variously struggled with joblessness, homelessness, loneliness, and abject poverty. I have come to consider my participants' willingness to let me into their space and their day-to-day lives for those hours to be an extraordinary gift—one that, I hope, will help scholars understand how speakers with diagnoses of chronic mental conditions and other stigmatized, vulnerable persons utilize compelling appeals to *ethos* and display flexible episteme when they interact with each other, with outsiders, and with their care providers.

Coding: Recuperative *Ethos* and Agile Epistemologies

Participants in my study demonstrated nostalgic regard for lost credibility. In fact, as I note above, one of the major terms I developed to characterize their everyday talk is "recuperative *ethos*," or the appeals woven into their day-to-day interactions that indicate they are worthwhile and reliable speakers, thinkers, lovers, friends, and community members. As examples of ephemeral rhetorical performance, appeals to recuperative *ethos* represent the varied strategies through which rhetors diagnosed with severe mental illnesses establish *ethos* in the wake of highly stigmatizing illness experiences. Appeals to recuperative *ethos* also constitute speakers' attempts to mitigate the unrelenting losses with which they have had to contend following acute phases of illness.[7]

Alongside recuperative *ethos*, however, my participants exhibited extraordinary epistemic capacities. I characterize these moments as "agile epistemologies" to capture the way they productively disrupt underestimations of these orators' rhetorical abilities. In fact, agile epistemologies might be read as the residual effects of the very conditions that have left participants trying to recover credibility in the first place.[8] While describing the participants' appeals to *ethos* came easily, agile epistemologies were predictably more cumbersome data, which also made them fascinating.

In defining these related terms, Mol's notion of ontologies as emergent in the present became crucial. For Mol, understanding the complexities inherent in the multiple and shifting day-to-day performances that comprise a condition's nonlinear trajectory means gleaning the layers of being at play in the construction of the present. Recuperative *ethos* takes up the threads of credibility that weave in and out of everyday talk. Agile epistemologies take up the idea of neurodiversity as generative affordance in order to suggest that mental illnesses, while stigmatizing and undeniably damaging to rhetorical *ethos*, come with certain rhetorical advantages. Agile epistemologies, moreover, unfold in the data beyond the kinds of poetic tropes common in published works of fiction, memoirs, and the like. Likewise, as forms of vernacular rhetoric, recuperative *ethos* and agile epistemologies are "always operating in the background, reflecting how social actors understand and participate in the constriction of their world" (Hauser, 2011, p. 166).

As Chapter 1 made clear, contemporary rhetoricians complicate "*ethos*" in order to render its analyses and its uses more sensitive to socially complex contexts, and I made use of their contributions in coding.[9] Scholars especially address the binary separating theories of *ethos* as embedded in the moment of oratorical performance versus *ethos* as constructed via the demographic and institutional realities that supersede the oratorical scene. Jarratt (2002) explained, for instance, that Aristotle's definition of *ethos* leaves readers to imagine the "rhetorical scene as two-dimensional" and as "fixed in the moment of rhetorical performance" (p. 30). Amossy (2001) described *ethos* as both "constructed within verbal interactions" and "inscribed in a symbolic exchange governed by social mechanisms and external institutional positions" (p. 5). *Ethos* is, thus, always a combination of the past and the present and of the relatively fixed and the ephemeral. Amossy (2001) also pointed out how speakers tend to the "construction of image" in the context of "stereotypes" the "target public" might hold (p. 7). For Amossy (2001), *ethos* is a speaker's engagement with the transaction between who they are at the inception of oratorical performance and what these demographic and institutionally driven shades of self make available for that performance.

Similarly, Reynolds (1993) pointed out that work on *ethos* might more usefully be described as having the potential to "open up more spaces in which to study writers' subject positions or identity formations, especially to examine how writers establish authority and enact responsibility from positions not traditionally considered authoritative" (p. 326). These scholars suggest the need to examine how one establishes credibility when she or he is in a position of disenfranchisement. Using this lens, I categorized the speech acts of participants as potentially working in direct refutation to the stigma that rendered their credibility questionable. These scholars, then, open space for thinking about how a speaker imagines and works against the audience's probable or stated perception, which is useful for coding data collected from a highly stigmatized population.

Likewise, rhetoricians interested in RHM have paved the way for studies that make use of *ethos* for granular analyses of everyday discursive performances.[10] Relying on verbatim speech acts from field notes and from transcriptions from audio-recordings, I developed the term "recuperative *ethos*" as a fitting descriptor of the appeals to *ethos* participants used, since "to recuperate" is to "recover a loss," or " to restore something to its original condition" (*OED Online*). After severe mental illness experiences, many participants lost quite a lot that they would naturally want to regain, such as lucrative and fulfilling employment, comfortable dwellings, desirable intimate partners, and a supportive network of family and friends. The rhetorical appeals I observed, therefore, appeared to be related to stigma and its consequences.

I developed the term "agile epistemologies" in order to account for data that appeared to be discursive habits at least partially born of so-called mentally "ill" ways of knowing.[11] That is, participants' everyday epistemologies seemed to be woven with the rich and interesting affordances of neurodiversity.[12] Agile bodies, of course, move with dexterity; agile minds "think, understand, and react quickly" (*OED Online*). Agile epistemologies are intriguing, inventive vernacular rhetorical performances that evoke an embodied experience of nimbleness. Moreover, as epistemologies, these quick-witted utterances performed meaning-making through language and gestures.

I developed the schema below to classify the forms of recuperative *ethos* and agile epistemologies that emerged in the data. Recuperative *ethos* include: displays of astuteness, arguments for strong human connections, and uses of religious *topoi*. Agile epistemologies include: logical contradiction, metonymic parallels, enthymemes, and expansive views on human agency. The coding scheme is described in Figure 5.1. In the following sections, I offer selected examples to illustrate where I located these appeals to recuperative *ethos* and forms of agile epistemologies in the data.

Recuperative *Ethos*: Displays of Astuteness	Recuperative *Ethos*: Strong Human Connections	Recuperative *Ethos*: Religious Topoi	Agile Epistemologies
• Expressions of social insight	• Descriptions of self as moral and empathetic	• Correspondence with god and god's interventions	• Logical contradiction
• Displays of experiential knowledge	• References to successful interpersonal relationships	• One's interpretive capabilities of religious and mystical texts and ideas	• Metonymic parallels
• References to book and scholarly knowledges		• Meaningful engagement with religious institutions	• Enthymemes
			• Notable views of human agency

Figure 5.1 Coding Scheme for Ethnographic Study of Mental Health

Recuperative *Ethos* via Displays of Astuteness

I have identified and coded three types of displays of astuteness in the data: expressions of social insight, displays of experiential knowledge, and references to book and scholarly knowledges. In some of its forms, displays of astuteness resemble Aristotle's (1991) account of practical knowledge in the *Rhetoric*. These displays of astuteness also rely on *phronesis* since they include assertion of practical wisdom born of social insight or experience. Moreover, participants rely on forms of knowledge that are regularly rewarded in contemporary American culture, such as book and scholarly knowledge, to argue for their astuteness. In a sense, displays of astuteness rely on *ethos* as one shade of the "significant force of rhetoric in engendering trust or suspicion in . . . public life" (Keränen, p. 3).

I define social insight as speakers' references to experiences in which they have been able to decode complex situations due to acute ability to quickly decipher unpredictable human behavior. To illustrate, when my participant John, a middle-aged African American man with a booming voice and infectious laugh, described his work with the task force meant to resolve clubhouse grievances to a clubhouse staff member, he explained the need to use one's instincts when facts are missing. Indeed, John suggested that he is quite adept at using this particular skill set. As he explained, it is important to think through what both sides of an argument have to say, especially when there are factual mismatches in opposing parties' accounts. Describing situations where two sides of a story display a contradiction, John said that one must ask, "Is it really this, or is it really *this*?" Thus, John replaced the traditional "that" in the latter segment of his utterance to suggest, perhaps, that it can be both; he suggests that the truth is often a gray area with multiple possibilities. In these circumstances, John remarked, "You have to really *think*." He explained that he is better able to handle these ambiguous situations since staff members are often looking for the definitive truth of a situation, while he is able to parse the complexity of social conflicts.

John is, likewise, proud of the fact that he has been able to use this ability to understand complex social circumstances to clear up many misunderstandings before they go to the higher authorities for whom, he insists, conflicts seem more difficult to resolve. He described, "Um, many times . . . we get both sides together and we try to resolve it before it goes any further." John credits his ability to, as he put it, "think beyond he-said-she-said" for his reputable work on the task force, and in this way seems to make an implicit argument for himself as possessing an insightful social intelligence.

In a related way, I define expressions of experiential knowledge as reminders for interlocutors of the participants' valuable sets of life experiences—incidences from which they have undergone significant personal growth and out of which they have gotten new forms of knowledge that would be otherwise inaccessible. The kinds of experiential knowledge woven into participants' conversations include references to illnesses (psychological and otherwise), including discussions of hospitalization and recovery; experiences working and spending leisure time at the clubhouse; and experiences at other places of employment, including, in some cases, working in the positions obtained through the clubhouse.

Referencing his military background, for example, my participant Bill, a tall and striking African American man, explained that killing, he knows "from experience," is a "real pleasure." As he told another participant, "Before you take a life, it's better than sex. You salivate. Believe me." This utterance might seem to be a strange example of recuperative *ethos* as admitting to having killed other people might further damage *ethos*. However, upon further analysis, it seems clear that Bill wishes to impart his world-wary position as one who has seen the darkest there is to see in humanity and who has, therefore, emerged as acutely sensitive to the contours of human nature—a sentiment he imparts implicitly through this job-related experience. Without this experience, he implied, a person cannot make any viable claims to know what it is to be fully and dauntingly human. In the same way, Bill's nighttime cab driver position entitles him to street credibility. He knows about the "seedy" sorts who take cabs in the middle of the night. He can handle these types, he assures listeners, although many others might not be willing or able to do so.

Participants also attempt to establish *ethos* with references to book and scholarly knowledge in two ways: through allusions to important texts and through descriptions of educational achievements. Segal (2003) explained that "in order to be taken as a reliable producer of natural knowledge" one must possess, among other things, a "mastery of a specialized theoretical vocabulary or experimental equipment, proper certification and institutional position" (p. 140). In the same way, speakers alluded to great works with which they are familiar or offered analyses of these with confidence. Participants also discussed their educational achievements and aspirations in order to highlight their intelligence, diligence, and ambition.

Stanley, a middle-aged white man, for instance, wishes to show that he is college-educated. Describing his time working toward a pharmacy technician certification, he remarked

> I mean, I, I was the top of the class, I do have a letter from Greenview Community College guidance department, they gave me a letter of recommendation, I was in the 75th percentile of the class, and I was leading the class, and, um, even during final examinations, the final exam, I did very well.[13]

He seemed proud to share that he learned practical information on this exam, such as "knowing the generics, the brand, uh, changing mic—micrograms into milligrams, the piggyback IV, um, there's, there, there were several things on the final exam." Through reiterating the specialized pharmaceutical knowledge needed to score so high on the exam, he showed listeners that his learning experiences in college were extensive, moving him beyond everyday knowledge on an important topic.

In each case, participants threaded indications of their astuteness, their social intelligences and educational achievements, their knowledge of great works, and their ability to incisively unpack esoteric content into their everyday conversations. Since they have been diagnosed with illnesses that affect the brain, and since pharmaceutical interventions are known to cloud thinking, they want to convince listeners of their exceptional intelligence. Thus, these appeals to *ethos* are similar to patients' use of high-quality research activities to bolster their credibility as discussed in Chapter 3.

Recuperative *Ethos* via Strong Human Connections

One particularly damaging stereotype of severe mental illness is that it renders a person unable to maintain meaningful relationships,[14] and participants countered this stigma via references to strong human connections. I coded two distinct types of this form of recuperative *ethos*: indications that they are moral and empathetic, and references to the successful inter-personal relationships they maintain. Stigma suggests that those with mental illness diagnoses do not have the capacity to decipher, let alone act according to, moral codes. These sorts of sentiments are reiterated each time a television character on a crime drama or, perhaps more impor-tantly, an actual human offender is deemed "not guilty" of a particularly heinous crime "by reasons of insanity." In these instances, "insanity" func-tions as a state in which a person's moral compass has been incapacitated. John put it best when he explained the damage done by the "poor portray-als" on the "shows that sensationalize" the experiences of persons with mentally illnesses wherein a character has a mental illness, and "Boom!" the narrative implies, "That gives him the right to kill." These depictions lead to people getting what John describes as "negative perceptions of the mental health community." He continued, "Even, like, if you see, like, in the newspaper, you always see, a lot of people read that . . . the mental health community is portrayed as someone portrayed in a crime. And then they say, 'Send them to Lakeview[15] for observation,' so a lot of people, all they see is that, and they get scared." John understands that fictional and nonfictional accounts of mental illnesses inspire fear when they emphasize the inability of persons with mental illness diagnoses to read the implicit cultural script for morally acceptable behavior.

For similar reasons, John is aware that mentally ill persons are regu-larly accused of lacking human empathic skills. In a clear instance of this capacity, John remarked, in reference to his work with his peers, "They've been hospitalized, um, so we know what they've gone through and what their struggles are in a hospital situation, so they have struggles in there, and we know what it's like, so they can relate to us better than to a doc-tor." John continued, "We hear a lot of their stories, and I get touched by some of the things I hear, um, from alcohol abuse, some people get battered, um, some people have cutting problems like I've had, and, from the background that they come from, it makes me want to help out and reach out and, even if it's just one person—it makes a world of difference to me." Clearly, John's choice to discuss these personal details and his outreach work reflects his knowledge of my status as clubhouse outsider. Still, these utterances likely mirror others through which John constructs *ethos* with various outsiders in his day-to-day life.

In another example of an empathic display, my fieldnotes document the following: A young woman I call Shakita sits at the hospitality unit's main table drinking coffee and sharing photos of her children. Gene, another participant, arrives; he slips through the back door looking disheveled and distressed. He lurks on the periphery of other conversations for some time. He is sort of slinking about leaning against a wall when Shakita calls him over. She greets him when he approaches and asks him how he is doing, and he says, with admirable honesty, "Not good." Shakita asks him what is wrong, and he says that he does not have any way to get to work because he does not have the bus fare. He asked his dad to lend it to him, but his dad told him, "I need to hold on to *my* money." Shakita smiles, "You're short, and believe me, I know how that feels, I got you for today. How much is it?"

He asks her, shamefacedly, if she can spare sixty cents, and she counts it out in nickels and pennies from her small change purse into his open palm. The coins flash from hand to hand. Gene is visibly relieved, and his day would be complete, he says, "if only [I] had a coffee," but he does not have fifty cents to get one from the snack bar. Shakita produces a Ziploc bag of instant coffee that she has brought in for herself. She buys two ten-cent paper cups from the snack bar and splits the instant coffee in two, which makes both cups rather thin and watery. He looks genuinely relieved, happy and taken care of, but Shakita whispers, "I hope he has food for later."

Another member overhears Shakita and gives Gene a piece of her Rice Krispies Treat. Gene pulls small sections from the treat and washes them down with his coffee. "I used to be eating plates like this" (he makes a large oval with his hands) "but then I switched to plates like this." He narrows the oval considerably. "In the house where I have a room, no one eats healthy. They eat all kind of meat, but not really any grains or nothing. I had used to eat collards and rice and chicken, and now . . .," but Gene does not finish. His voice trails off. He stares into his coffee.

In fact, over the course of observations, Gene will recall, in great detail, several meals eaten out in the past few years, and he will pay particular attention to portion, price and quality. The most piercing memory he shares is of a birthday several years past. On that day, he explained,

> It was pay day, and me and my friends, we had a few bucks, so we all, we took twenty bucks or so, and we had went to Applebee's, see, and I got me a huge plate, you know them really big plates that are like oval? And the whole bottom, it was covered in French fries, and the whole top, with, what you call them? Boneless ribs. And I was so, so full, I had drank a beer, too, so I was nice and full and I was nice and buzzed, you know, and I said to my friends, let's go to the beach and dance.

After he recalled this story, his smile broadened momentarily before fading out.

"They got a Chinese restaurant down in New York," Gene tells a table full of eager listeners, "And you gonna pay, maybe twenty or thirty bucks for a plate, but it's going to be a huge oval plate and it's gonna be covered, I mean *covered*, in food." His spectators nod in admiration. These members expressed their solidarity for the suffering Gene experiences in coming up short on money and food by eagerly listening to his stories of other times in which he has not suffered from such deprivation. Shakita, more importantly, demonstrated her ability to empathize—something that would be contested in clinical settings and various documents where her particular illness is described.[16]

Displays of important familial and other essential human connections are also significant components of recuperative *ethos*. In some ways, these appeals to *ethos* resemble the "credibility proxy" as discussed in Chapter 3. I have defined recuperative *ethos* through references to "close relationships" as places in conversation where speakers highlight their ability to be worthwhile intimate partners, family members, or friends. These expressions show interlocutors that the speaker is fully capable of making meaningful, loyal, and lasting personal commitments. Likewise, "close relationships" designates speakers' stated affiliations with those in positions of power—persons whose positive *ethos* is assumed by virtue of their standing. This rhetorical move might be meant to offset the negative *ethos* associated with a speaker's own institutional status as clubhouse member.[17]

Shakita, for instance, made a claim for her reliability when she described the man she was to marry as loyal and loving. Attracting such a mate is a sign of personal success, she implied. She also recounted his reaction to her choice to name their son after her brother. "I thought he was going to be mad. I named my, um, son after my brother, and I—he was like, 'No, I'm not mad at all,' he was like, 'I know how close you are with your brother.'" Before his untimely death, this responsible man had held a full-time job and had purchased a home for his young family. Since this fair, understanding, evenhanded person wanted to devote his life to her, Shakita frequently reminded peers of his admirable qualities in everyday conversations in order to reinforce her own self-worth in her listeners' eyes. Significantly, the fact that this admirable person is not in Shakita's life now is not her fault, nor is it due to her illness. As she explained, his life was "taken from him," and otherwise they would have been "married all this time."

Stanley frequently remarked that he has been invited by the mayor to attend an important event, and John threaded references to his various relationships with clubhouse staff and leadership into conversations with his peers, with other staff and leadership, and with outsiders. Through references to intimate relations with admirable qualities and to relationships with institutionally sanctioned leaders, participants attempt to recover their own damaged *ethos*. Far from the symptoms checklists and other documents that discursively construct some of their diagnoses, participants made it clear, in day-to-day life, that they are valuable, desirable social actors capable of complex, rich social lives. If they have been left behind, as many have been by family, friends, and acquaintances, it is not because they are not worthwhile. These everyday arguments for credibility are sharp reminders of the savage injustices of stigma: it often leaves highly vulnerable persons without community at their lowest points.

Recognizing their damaged *ethos*, these participants made similar moves to those described in Chapter 3 as using a "credibility proxy" wherein another person's stronger *ethos* is strategically attached to the speaker by association.

Recuperative *Ethos* via Religious *Topoi*

Pryal (2010) explained that mood memoirists (authors with mood disorders narrating their illness stories) use various rhetorical tactics in order to establish an *ethos* that might work against stigma and "rhetorical exclusion" via "political counter-narratives to the dominant psychiatric narratives about mental illness" (p. 483). Absent from her compelling analysis are the intricate store of everyday, rhetorically driven, religious and mystical topics-as-invention on which my participants rely in order to recuperate damaged *ethos*. These *topoi* rely quite heavily on clubhouse *doxa* since, like other institutions where lives are being rebuilt, there is a strong religious undercurrent to day-to-day life there. Three main religious and mystical topics that seem to be part of recuperative *ethos* for the participants emerged in my analysis: 1) correspondence with god and god's interventions in one's life as indication of a purposeful existence; 2) interpretive capabilities of religious and mystical texts, including knowledge of religious, mystical, or morals-based aphorisms and clichés; and 3) meaningful engagement with religious institutions. Each of these topics overlaps with two main themes: "absolute knowledge of god's existence" and "the value in suffering."

The *topos* "god's intervention in one's life" includes those utterances wherein a speaker articulates her or his own importance in human history, which they substantiate by direct or oblique reference to the will of a higher power. In these statements, speakers attempt to demonstrate God's decision to intervene and to answer prayers, thus tacitly arguing for self-worth; Bill's comments on his relationship to the divine is a strong example of this *topos*.

"God would not let me go," Bill mutters between drags of his cigarette that create an ethereal smokescreen dividing him from Shakita. Bill would have gladly given up life rather than endure as he has. A divine hand is at work in the world, Bill suggests, and this force believes Bill's existence to be not only worthwhile, but essential. Bill made it clear that he has made very real attempts to end his life, ones that would have certainly killed other people. Through emphasizing the miraculous nature of his survival and god's will inherent in this continued existence, Bill argued that he has, to god's mind, an extraordinary role to fulfill here on earth. Thus, by acknowledging his suicide attempts, Bill displayed a strong and resilient character impervious to existential fears. He manages, in this fashion, to humbly describe himself as above average in the eyes of the divine.

The unlikely rhetor's exceptional interpretive capacity regarding religious and mystical texts and phenomena are also apparent in the data. This *topos*, which involves speakers drawing on assertions of a deeper-than-average ability to distill complicated metaphysics for less sensitive audiences, has thematic links to both the certain knowledge of god's existence and an afterlife as well as to the value of suffering. To illustrate, Bill explained the "truth" of spirituality to Shakita one afternoon, which, he asserted, he knows well, as he has read and interpreted "every version of the Bible and the Koran, and they are all the same."

"The Koran," he tells her, "is the same as the Old Testament of the Bible," and Shakita noticeably exhales with relief when Bill passes on this revelation. Interestingly, she does not question its accuracy for a moment. Bill has managed to communicate a complicated insight—that all religious texts, even those that serve as charter documents for disparate religious institutions—communicate the same messages from the divine. In fact, Bill's argument here follows a similar logical trajectory as Latour's (1999) in *Pandora's Hope*, where he demonstrated that all forms of expert knowledge, even those that appear to be at odds, serve the same function: to shut out the masses and to keep their voices silent. Bill's tone is not exactly conspiratorial, though. Instead, he attempts to show Shakita that religious texts all convey essentially the same messages from god, and these messages are at odds with their articulations in various institutions (specifically in their antagonism toward each other). Bill seems to be onto something important: that there is a remarkable sameness to dogmatic religious expression. Bill, thus, displayed a keen eye toward similar messages being codified in starkly different ways.

At the conclusion of Bill's explanation, Shakita replied, blithely, "Oh! I always wondered what the difference was, and now I know!" She looked admiringly at Bill; he looked past her. Shakita's facial expressions and tone indicated that she was not only being polite. Instead, it seemed clear that she was convinced that Bill possessed the interpretive capacity to make such a strong claim—one that she seemed sure was irrefutable. Through his elaborate analysis of biblical texts, Bill's attempt to bolster his *ethos* was largely successful.

Clubhouse members Veronica and Gretchen also showcased their approaches to human life as a temporary and mostly arduous and passive waiting period for the better place to come. They did so in their uses of religiously inspired aphorisms, such as Gretchen's assertion that "God is everywhere." In the same way, when the women hear someone from a far-off room curse: "Oh my Lord Jesus!" Gretchen replies swiftly with, "That's who we need, is Jesus." The women clearly equate goodness and heavenly rewards with plainly stated belief in god and in Jesus, along with participation of some kind in "church." Shortly after I met them, Veronica explained plainly, "We both go to church." In the end, Gretchen explained, "[we are] god's children," and we suffer on earth so that we might end up "in a better place."

In each datum included in religious and mystical *topoi*, speakers fold religious and mystical themes into conversations to strengthen their *ethos*. My participants lost jobs, intimate partners, the support of family and friends, and their standing in their communities after especially severe episodes involving hallucinations, delusions, and, ultimately, hospitalization. Through recuperative *ethos* via religious *topoi*, speakers attempt to regain the credibility that they feel has been lost following the onset, diagnosis, and treatment of severe mental illness by implying that their experiences are all part of god's plan and that they are better prepared for spiritual challenges because of them. The clubhouse—a liminal space meant to buffer the time between hospitalization and/or acute illness experiences and a more stable future—was a site where this particular form of *ethos* was especially prevalent.

Agile Epistemologies

I coded data "agile epistemologies" when participants' engagement with language might have been drawing on the rhetorical affordances that accompany their conditions. In these interchanges, participants exhibited the poetic and arresting linguistic affordances regularly attributed to diverse ways of knowing born of so-called mental illnesses conceived broadly,[18] but here they unfold in proliferative, multiple ways that suggest the intricate ontologies at play at the clubhouse. In order to organize these discursive behaviors systematically, I catalogued the types that seemed, in the moment, to shift perspectives or to showcase cognitive dexterity. These included: logical contradiction, metonymic parallels, enthymemes, and expansive views of human agency. Participants expressed concern for people prying into their stories of acute-mental-illness-related experiences when we went through informed consent. It occurred to me that, too often, those with severe mental illness diagnoses are encouraged to do just that—to write out their stories, to seek a voice. Indeed, the anti-stigma campaigns discussed in Chapter 2 largely operate under the assumption that getting those with mental illness diagnoses to share their stories is an effective way to fight stigma. However, I found participants to be rightly guarded against this outcome, as they perceived researchers' interests in their stories akin to, as participant Mel put it, "making them guinea pigs." Thus, in the end, my analysis displays a rich array of potent everyday rhetorics that do not necessarily draw on deeply personal and/or traumatic anecdotes for expressive or cathartic ends.

I coded instances in which logical contradictions made an impact on a listener as examples of agile epistemologies. To illustrate, one morning Gene's staff leader admonished him since he had been skipping his therapy appointments. If he did not resume these sessions, she said, his housing assistance would be terminated. Gene countered confidently, "If they take my housing away, I'm not going to have anywhere to live, so I'll have to leave this state." The staff leader looked genuinely perplexed. She began to stammer a bit and to offer Gene some alternatives: he could get a new therapist or adjust the schedule of appointments to better suit his needs. Here, Gene's syntax indicated that he believed (and, more importantly, asserted) that his housing is the only possible place for him to live in the city where the clubhouse is located. Further, he is arguing that the homelessness that could result from his missed psychiatric appointments cannot follow him elsewhere. This is a powerful moment in Gene's everyday speech, representing his attempt to regain authority when he feels he is being backed into a corner. He is trying to redistribute the power dynamic between himself and his staff leader, and he is somewhat successful. His listener is utterly confused by the syntactical structure of his logic, which is probably because it is happening in real time and not in writing, where she would have been able to think through the fallacious nature of his claim and would not have had the burden of needing to reply quickly. In this example, Gene proves capable of some unlikely, though powerful, rhetorical agility in everyday talk.

The items I describe as metonymic parallels with critical overlays are instances in which a speaker infuses the description of some unrelated matter with the energy one might assume belongs to another. The former reference, though, is only a matter of analytic conjecture, as that which is substituted remains unnamed. In this way, metonymic parallels with critical overlays resemble Cintron's (2003) analysis of a T-shirt he took to be symbolic in a participant he observed in his ethnographic research. As he explains, "I cannot know the intentions of the manufacturer or the wearer. Nevertheless, I think the T-shirt was consistent with a larger set of neighborhood meanings" (p. 33). Although it is debatable whether or not speakers intend for these uses to be understood this way, these elaborate structures rely on highly complex and coherent metonymics in which one issue relationally references another. These utterances, which are likely discernable in other populations, "could indicate a time not captured by the literal meaning of the words but by their context" (Hauser, 2011, p. 157). There is even a sense, in some exchanges, that listeners understand the speaker to be referencing one set of emotive experiences via a less contentious description of another. As such, these instances might have been read as euphemistic, but there is a messier relationship between sign and signifier than euphemism allows (hence the inherent agility). As discursive behavior is always a manifestation of something else—identity, social constructions, cognition, and the like—perhaps readers will suspend disbelief momentarily and consider the following examples.

Over the course of data collection, Shakita shared with me and with many of her clubhouse friends her plans to get a pet cockatiel. She mentioned the books and websites she'd read and the people she had consulted about how to care for these lovely, delicate creatures "correctly." She was sure, though, that the way to care for *her* bird would not require following exactly what the owner's guides and pet-store workers have told her. Shakita wanted to take care of this cockatiel, but she insisted that she did not "want to put a cover over the cage."

"They say you have to put a cover over the cage so that the bird will know when it is supposed to sleep," she explained to a table full of hospitality unit members before the morning meeting, "but it will sleep when it's tired, and I am not going to scare it by covering up its cage." While some members expressed confusion and concern over the fact that Shakita intended to flout expert cockatiel care advice, when she explained this matter to Bill, he looked at her with a knowing smile and nodded while pointing several times at her as if to say, "You've got it!" What might alert listeners like Bill to the multiple meanings Shakita likely intended here is the contradiction at the heart of her incessant seeking out of expert knowledge. She had been, as she explained, "preparing" to own this creature for several months by reading books, consulting websites, and talking with the staff at the pet store from which she hopes, eventually, to procure the bird. However, when she recounted these experiences to others, the most important part of her narrative was not that she had learned all there was to know and was ready to take on this owner-ship. Instead, she emphatically stated that she intended not to follow these expert sources' most basic piece of advice on care: place the bird in a covered cage if you wish for it to sleep. One might say that Shakita, in repeating this line so many times and to so many listeners, wished to comment on the nature of expert knowledge when they take over a person's own critical capacity for thoughtful, humane conclusions. This analysis might be considered a stretch, of course, but it also recognizes "propriety within vernacular rhetoric," which "often manifests in a dis-course that implicitly critiques outsiders, usually official power" (Hauser, 2011, p. 165). Shakita dexterously weaves her critiques of limiting, hege-monic discourses into her everyday talk.

Hauser (2011) framed his assertion that "language in use always entails interrogation of power" and that the "speech of leaders is always at odds with that of those they seek to dominate" by employing Mikhail Bakhtin's concept of heteroglossia—"the diversity of unofficial forms of a national language" that "guarantees an utterance's meaning is a func-tion of its prevailing conditions of time and place" and Burke's asser-tion that humans act "through symbolic forms embedded in the everyday performance of social action" (p. 162). In a similar way, I find a poten-tial link between Shakita's comments on her cockatiel plans to a critique of the mental healthcare system and the clubhouse institution itself—especially since Shakita has been openly critical of the more formulaic and arbitrary-seeming rules governing clubhouse life.

For instance, a few months before I began my observation, Shakita told me, she had brought supplies to bake a cake to share with her friends, but was denied the use of the kitchen because the food was not purchased by kitchen staff members. Aptly, she pointed out that the clubhouse ideal that everyone feel at home is inconsistent with the strict rules regarding kitchen usage. Since openly criticizing the clubhouse would be a risky thing to do in the presence of clinical staff, Shakita shared the details of this event with me early one morning before many others had arrived. In contrast, the cockatiel story, since it is a coded way of criticizing rules, guidelines, and regulations that take strictness and procedures into account first, and human and creaturely needs second, can be shared frequently and publicly. Both cases make her agile episteme clear: she will not make decisions on how to treat other people or vulnerable creatures based solely on expert knowledge if her own, local knowledge and instincts tell her that there are better alternatives.

Enthymemes are a third type of agile epistemology I find in the data. Enthymemes, of course, rely on audience *doxa*. The participants' ruminations I discuss below are unique; they are syntactically structured as if the speaker believes that the starting premise of the utterance is an absolute and organically verifiable truth, such as, in the classic syllogism, "All men are mortal." However, traditional logic dictates that these starting points are actually probable, contingent, and mutable truths—the kinds of assertions more commonly associated with enthymemes. Bill's explanation, when he recalled his failed suicide attempts, that there is a part of the brain that will not let you die (as if it were a reverse Achilles tendon) functions this way as his utterance makes it clear that he believes this assertion to be organically irrefutable. In an everyday conversation with Shakita, this enthymeme is received exactly as if it were an absolute truth; Shakita does not appear to doubt its verifiability for one second.

In the same way, when Shakita lamented her strained relationship with her mother, Bill told her, "My father tries to tell me that I'm evil or crazy, but parents don't understand that if *we* are, then *they* are, 'cause we came from them." Shakita smiled. It seems significant here that Shakita finds the premise that makes up the first part of Bill's utterance to be irrefutably true; if she did not find it so, it is unlikely that she would have been quickly comforted by the remark. These enthymemes work with audiences precisely because they are stated as if they were syllogisms and are, thus, either received as such or are nimble enough to make a listener think the matter through more thoroughly.

Expansive views on human agency embedded into everyday talk were also coded as agile epistemologies. These views of human agency suggest that, contrary to the dominant culture's understanding of credentials and those who are authorized to offer new knowledge, anyone is capable of inventing and conveying meaning. An interesting incident occurred along these lines one afternoon at the snack bar. Maxwell was selling a cup of coffee to an elderly man who seemed to be almost completely nonverbal. The man gave Maxwell money for the coffee; Maxwell placed a Styrofoam coffee cup ceremoniously on the counter and carefully cupped the man's quivering, upturned palm in order to count out a small a pile of coins for change.

Kyle, meanwhile, looked on vigilantly with arms crossed over his chest and an uncharacteristically hostile scowl miring his ordinarily friendly face. The man gathered up his coffee with his free hand before shuffling over to Kyle to give him the coins. After the transaction was completed, Kyle erupted angrily, "I knew you were gonna fuck it up!" The man looked at the ground and let out a sort of whimper. Maxwell looked up with alarm in his eyes, but did not say anything as Kyle continued to rant: "I gave him a dollar and a quarter, and he was supposed to give me seventy-five cents change, but he only gave me fifty, but I knew he would fuck it up." I looked on stunned. A ruse, I suppose, but to prove what?

Maxwell did not offer a verbal reply, but responded, instead, by slowly opening the cash register. Gazing down, he handed Kyle a quarter. Maxwell's nonverbal reaction seemed to calm Kyle down a bit, which is perhaps why Kyle then told Maxwell, "I wasn't mad at you, I was just mad at him, because I *knew* he would fuck it up." Maxwell did not offer a rejoinder. Instead, he smiled weakly and picked up his dusting cloth to clear the counter. What is curious here is that a cup of coffee costs fifty cents (which Kyle knew), so Kyle's decision to give a friend a dollar and a quarter for a cup of coffee that costs only fifty cents seemed to have been a test of sorts.

This performative ruse was so seamlessly threaded into everyday life that it palpably disconcerted all social actors present in one way or another. Some onlookers stood deathly still during this exchange and for several seconds afterward. Most others hurried away like busy pedestrians clearing a sidewalk when the rain begins. They slid out the back door pretending to need a cigarette, or they speed-walked to the front units under the guise of pressing work. Kyle wanted to cause a disturbance, and he was successful in that aim.

Kyle's comment to Maxwell, moreover, made it is possible to read this situation as Kyle creating this instructive tableau of sorts in order to show onlookers that he was capable of predicting human behavior and that his own agency exceeded the ordinary. It seems that Kyle orchestrated this scenario, in other words, to show audiences that he was able to predict, or even to dictate, how others would act and react in certain situations. He was expressing superagency, which stands in stark contrast to the loss of control that is regularly attributed to those with mental illness diagnoses. More compelling, though, is his unusual and attention-grabbing way of symbolically showcasing this agency.

Recuperative *Ethos* and Agile Epistemologies as Generative Terms for RHM and MHRR

Emmons (2008) illustrated the value of rhetorical lenses for revealing troubling truths in well-intentioned mental healthcare and for articulating alternatives, especially in her robust discussions of depression as a gendered diagnosis, her treatment of patients' tendencies to "self-doctor" in response to pharmaceutically constructed versions of conditions, and in her description of a "rhetoric care of the self," which involves nurturing "the habits of critical reading and dialogic engagement with the discourses of health and illness" (p. 181). My participants demonstrated their rhetorical fitness for deliberative spaces fraught with the pervasive stigma against them; this stigma is well documented in social science research (see, for example, Hinshaw, 2007; Pescosolido et al., 2010). Most pressing for rhetoricians is the fact that stigma takes potential rhetors out of the polis altogether and renders them less-than-fully-human. An individual with a mental illness diagnosis, then, is not only attempting to establish credibility, but is attempting to dig out of a rhetorical black hole.

Prendergast (2001) asked whether or not "there will ever be a rhetoric of mental disability that the mentally disabled themselves will have the greatest part in crafting" (p. 59). Rhetoricians have made significant strides in documenting the formidable landscape that constitutes the social and discursive construction of medicine, health, and wellness in recent years. One strand of this scholarship attempts to create "a genre of research that seeks to contribute to clinical work," which is not meant to prove that particular practices are right or wrong, but to "contribute to improving them" by "unraveling" the "tensions that people, both professionals and patients, live with" (Mol, 2000, p. 411). As I hope this chapter makes clear, there is much to be learned from studying everyday rhetorical performances in clinical and other institutional settings when it comes to the tensions with which vulnerable people live.

A focus on vernacular rhetoric alongside a focus on the multiple ontologies at play in these sites offers fertile grounds from which generative new theoretical concepts might emerge. Beyond theories of persuasion, though, are the promising lines of inquiry made available in rhetorical scholarship focusing on how we increasingly construct our sense of selves around biological categories at the expense of a much richer repertoire (Berkenkotter, 2008; Segal, 2005). Thus, the rhetorical performances I describe in this chapter illustrate two concepts that might fruitfully be applied to other cases in RHM and beyond. They offer a glimpse of how ordinary people work against stigma and diagnostic criteria in their everyday lives.

Kleinman (2013) argued that more primacy ought to be given to "the social suffering that affects everyone, but especially marginalized people already injured by poverty, isolation, and other forms of structural violence" (p. 1377). Vulnerable and stigmatized persons, of course, are over-represented among those Kleinman (1988) described. More than others, they need to be heard. The concepts of recuperative *ethos* and agile epistemologies offer preeminence to these marginalized people's varied ways of being by naming, parsing, and analyzing what otherwise might be throwaway. They offer a site of praxis through which we might offer solace to such persons by honoring what they are offering. In this way, the concepts might usefully inform scholarship examining the everyday rhetorical performances of other vulnerable, stigmatized populations such as those in prisons, hospices, intensive care units, and homeless shelters.

Cintron (1993) argued that field-based methods in rhetoric possess the "potential to encounter radically new information" (p. 406). The information that could be gathered in diverse sites using recuperative *ethos* and agile epistemologies as framing mechanisms—heuristics even—could be radical indeed. Moreover, through fragments of how stigmatized persons use rhetorical performances in their day-to-day lives, through glimpses of how they are trying to manage to be persuasive, much can be learned about how to better serve these individuals. Hauser and McClellan (2009) argued "that moment-by-moment interactions in the street, as well as sustained discourse among ordinary citizens" has the capacity to get at the "resistance found in seemingly mundane expressions" (25). This chapter answers their provocation with data and analyses that focus on under-investigated forms of being as they unfold in real time. Here, in this chapter, are analyses that focus on how everyday utterances, if taken seriously, might also be taken as meaningful. These terms introduced, moreover, highlight how stigmatized persons attempt to reclaim their places in the world and how they use displays of their unique attributes to resist those who would leave them behind.

Recuperative *ethos* and agile epistemologies constitute valuable conceptual resources for subsequent scholarship in RHM in its various forms. Protected populations are often stigmatized, with stigma leading to *ethos* deficit, damage, or loss. The sheer tenacity of the human spirit means that everyday people suffering from the menacing effects of stigmas use language to push back against this force. In doing so, speakers likely harness something uncommon in terms of rhetorical ability from the very differences for which that stigma unfairly follows them. Recuperative *ethos* and agile epistemologies also acknowledge the value of this population's ephemeral language practices, which are often ignored or dismissed as the residue of inchoate symptoms and not worth parsing, precisely because they lack narrative content or structure. It is my hope that future scholarship will be able to make use of and sharpen the definitions of these terms and that their continued refinement is informed by everyday talk from diverse participants who would otherwise remain unheard. Like the related studies that make up this book, this study engages very thorny and difficult-to-access human health issues that are already being addressed in other scholarship where the health sciences and humanities intersect. Like those studies that take up stigma, self-stigma, and recovery, this study comes into contact with deeply troubling socioeconomic realities. For now, this study presents a menagerie of vernacular rhetorics that clarify some of the multiple ontologies at play in the lived experiences of mental illnesses. As John would put it, this kind of work could "make a world of difference."

Researchers Megan Thorvilson and Adam Copeland (2018) adapted the concept of "recuperative *ethos*" in their essay "Incompatible with Care: Examining Trisomy 18 Medical Discourse and Families' Counter-discourse for Recuperative *Ethos*"—an essay published in the *Journal of Medical Humanities*. These scholars adapt and extend the terms to bring unique insight into complex health and medical contexts. In the same way, Miller (2019) used recuperative *ethos* to discuss Chris Christie's efforts to recover credibility that had been unfairly damaged due to his status as obese. These innovative adaptations of recuperative *ethos* show the value of pliable theoretical contributions in rhetoric and their capacity to inform and enrich future study.

Notes

1. This chapter is derived, in part, from an article published in *Rhetoric Society Quarterly* on April 3, 2015, available online: www.tandfonline.com/doi/abs/10.1080/02773945.2015.1010125.
2. Pescosolido and colleagues (2010) also explain that those working in public health have a vested interest in ending stigma, since it leads to fewer individuals with mental illnesses seeking care.
3. Self-stigma refers to conditions in which a member of a stigmatized group is "aware of" and "agrees with" negative stereotypes (Mittal et al., 2012, p. 974).
4. Prendergast (2001) aptly describes this tension when she points out that her acknowledgment of schizophrenia as a brain disease puts her "on a collision course with many of [her] colleagues with whom [she] generally shares . . . a number of basic epistemological assumptions," as she, too, has "generally poststructuralist leanings," which make her admissions that schizophrenia is a disease "sound at best conservative and at worst theoretically unsound" (p. 47).
5. In many ways, my project resembles what others have called "rhetorical ethnography" (Cintron, 2003; Cintron, 1993; Conquergood, 1992; Sangren, 1988). These studies, explains Cintron (2003), relied on the fact "that rhetorical analysis can help make sense of everyday language use," and that "rhetorical analysis need not be about famous speeches and/or the written word. Indeed, it need not be about the discursive at all and should also include the non-discursive and performative" (p. 5). These studies are valuable since rhetorical ethnography is often on a "collision course search for outlandish data that unsettle familiar truths" (Conquergood, 1992, p. 81). Ethnographic recounting, too, "can produce rich stories of lived bodies in which medicine figures as a part of daily life," and this kind of storytelling often involves "jagged story-lines . . . told by a variety of narrators whose voices may be drawn together and/or clash" (Mol & Law, 2004, p. 58). I, thus, call the project

"partly ethnographic," as Mol (2000) has described her own research (p. 82). Like Mol's work, what follows is "a hybrid genre"; it mixes "the philosophical aim of crafting theoretical terms with the practiographical style of telling stories" (Mol, 2000, p. 84).

6. Recruitment mechanisms and data collection procedures were designed in consult with the clubhouse director and the IRB as noninvasively as possible and as mostly observational—two characteristics that are hallmarks of naturalistic inquiry. The project went through full board review in July of 2010 and was approved after revisions on August 5, 2010, prior to data collection (study number 178158–2).

7. Recuperative *Ethos* might resemble other populations' *Ethos*-establishing appeals.

8. Even though they might be traceable in other populations.

9. With the affordances opened up by these rereadings of rhetorical *Ethos* and how it might be understood in contemporary contexts, Hyde (2004), for instance, in *The Ethos of rhetoric*, made a convincing case for a recovering the pre-Aristotelian sense of *Ethos* as dwelling place. Lisa Keränen (2010) examined *Ethos* in the context of scientists whose credibility has been compromised and how they attempt to recover *Ethos* via the strategic use of voice in the construction of persona. Cheng (2008) examined the construction of *Ethos* in an online educational chat; she concludes, "Through strategic positioning, evaluations, and stylistic choices, speakers portrayed their positive behavior, revealed personal values, and demonstrated individuality" (p. 223). Cheng (2008) asserted that her participants were able to "strengthen their *Ethos* by demonstrating qualities such as knowledge, competence, and authority appropriate to their profession" (p. 223).

10. For instance, in relation to how physicians and psychiatrists are trained to gain compliance from patients, Segal (2005) explained that what at first glance appears to be an appeal to *pathos* is actually an appeal to *Ethos*. Thus, if a patient suffers from issues related to obesity, a physician might try to identify with that patient by sharing a tendency to overeat, following it up with an indication that they overcome that tendency. For Segal, this scripted method "trades on" rather than "recalibrates" power dynamics between physicians and patients; thus, physicians engage "not in empathy but in moralism" (Segal, 2003, p. 137). Among her definitions, Segal (2005) defines *Ethos* as the "persuasiveness of the physician" (p. 152). I build on this work by suggesting the everyday ways in which a patient becomes persuasive or not via recuperative *Ethos* and agile epistemologies.

11. This is not to say that other populations do not use these tactics, but to say that the mental "illnesses" with which participants suffer might also generate rhetorical resources.

12. Although the term "neurodiversity" is most frequently used to describe neurological attributes of those on the autism spectrum (see, for example, the work of Ann Jurecic, 2007), it has also been used to describe the linguistic and cognitive affordances of those with other mental disorders and mental illnesses.

13. In order to protect anonymity, this community college name is fictional.

14. Many participants discussed how their mental health experiences and diagnoses led them to lose loved ones.

15. I have changed the name of the local psychiatric hospital to a fictional one in order to maintain participants' anonymity.

16. In many ways, these forms of recuperative *Ethos* resemble eunoia or goodwill as it is described in Aristotle's *Rhetoric* (see Aristotle, 1991). Shakita shared even more compelling references to her exceptional abilities to be moral and

empathetic, but these were exceedingly private things she chose to disclose that she explicitly asked me not to share with readers or anyone else.

17. Clubhouse members, of course, must have formal diagnoses of chronic mental illnesses to qualify for services.

18. For a thorough articulation of these, see Pryal (2010) and Horton (2013).

References

Amossy, R. (2001). *Ethos* at the crossroads of disciplines: Rhetoric, pragmatics, sociology. *Poetics Today, 22*(1), 1–23. doi:10.1215/03335372-22-1-1.

Angrosino, M. V. (2007). *Naturalistic observation.* Walnut Creek, CA: Left Coast Press. doi:10.1177/1049732310392593.

Aristotle. (1991). *On rhetoric: A theory of civic discourse* (G. A. Kennedy, Ed.). Oxford, UK: Oxford University Press.

Barker, P. (2003). The tidal model: Psychiatric colonization, recovery and the paradigm shift in mental healthcare. *International Journal of Mental Health Nursing, 12*(2), 96–102. doi:10.1046/j.1440-0979.2003.00275.x.

Berkenkotter, C. (2008). *Patient tales: Case histories and the uses of narrative in psychiatry.* Columbia, SC: University of South Carolina Press.

Britzman, D., & Pitt, A. J. (2004). Pedagogy and clinical knowledge: Some psychoanalytic observations on losing and refining significance. *JAC, 24*(2), 353–373.

Cassell, E. J. (1986). Ideas in conflict: The rise and fall (and rise and fall) of new views of disease. *America's Doctors, Medical Science, Medical Care, 115*(2), 19–41.

Cheng, M. (2008). *Ethos* and narrative in online educational chat. In B. Johnson & C. Eisenhart (Eds.), *Rhetoric in detail: Discourse analyses in rhetorical talk and text* (pp. 195–226). Philadelphia, PA: John Benjamins Publishing Company. doi:10.1075/dapsac.31.13che.

Cintron, R. (1993). Wearing a pith helmet at a sly angle: Or, can writing researchers do ethnography in a postmodern era? *Written Communication, 10*(3), 371–412. doi:10.1177/0741088393010003003.

Cintron, R. (2003). 'Gates locked' and the violence of fixation. In M. P. Nystrand & J. Duffy (Eds.), *Towards a rhetoric of everyday life: New directions in research on writing, text, and discourse* (pp. 5–37). Madison, WI: University of Wisconsin Press.

Conquergood, D. (1992). Ethnography, rhetoric, and performance. *Quarterly Journal of Speech, 78*(1), 80–97. doi:10.1080/00335639209383982.

Emmons, K. (2008). 'It's all in the uptake': Uptake in talk about depression. In B. Heifferon & S. C. Brown (Eds.), *Rhetoric of Healthcare* (pp. 159–180). Cresskill, NJ: Hampton Press.

Endres, D., Hess, A., Senda-Cook, S., & Middleton, M. K. (2016). In situ rhetoric. *Cultural Studies, Critical Methodologies, 16*(6), 511–524. doi:10.1177/1532708616655820.

Fardella, J. A. (2008). The recovery model: Ethics and the retrieval of the self. *Journal of Medical Humanities, 29*, 111–126. doi:10.1007/s10912-008-9054-4.

Hauser, G. A. (2011). Attending the vernacular: A plea for ethnographic rhetoric. In C. Meyer & F. Girke (Eds.), *The rhetorical emergence of culture* (pp. 157–172). New York: Berghahn.

Hauser, G. A., & McClellan, E. D. (2009). Vernacular rhetoric and social movements: Performances and resistance in the rhetoric of the everyday. In S. M.

Stevens & P. M. Malesh (Eds.), *Active voices: Composing a rhetoric of social movements* (pp. 23–46). Albany, NY: Suny University Press.

Hill, C. A. (2004). The psychology of rhetorical images. In C. A. Hill & M. Helmers (Eds.), *Defining visual rhetorics* (pp. 25–40), Mahwah, NJ: Erlbaum.

Hinshaw, S. D. (2007). *The mark of shame: Stigma of mental illness and an agenda for change.* Oxford, UK: Oxford University Press.

Holladay, D. (2017). Classified conversations: Psychiatry and tactical technical communication in online spaces. *Technical Communication Quarterly, 26*(1), 8–24. doi:10.1080/10572252.2016.1257744.

Horton, S. S. (2013). *Affective disorder and the writing life: The melancholic muse.* London, UK: Palgrave. doi:10.1057/9781137381668.

Hyde, M. (2004). *The ethos of rhetoric.* Columbia, SC: University of South Carolina Press.

Jarratt, S. (2002). Sappho's memory. *Rhetoric Society Quarterly, 32*(1), 11–43. doi:10.1080/02773940209391219.

Johnson, J. (2010). The skeleton on the couch: The Eagleton affair, rhetorical disability, and the stigma of mental illness. *Rhetoric Society Quarterly, 40*(5), 459–478. doi:10.1080/02773945.2010.517234.

Jurecic, A. (2007). Neurodiversity. *College English, 69*(5), 421–442. doi:10.2307/25472229.

Keränen, L. (2010). *Scientific characters: Rhetoric, politics, and trust in breast cancer research.* Tuscaloosa, AL: University of Alabama Press. doi:10.1080/02773945.2012.707964.

Kleinman, A. (1988). *The illness narratives: Suffering, healing and the human condition.* New York: Basic Books. doi:10.1097/ACM.0000000000001864.

Kleinman, A. (2013). From illness as culture to caregiving as moral experience. *New England Journal of Medicine, 368*(15), 1376–1377. doi:10.1056/NEJMp1300678.

Latour, B. (1999). *Pandora's hope: Essays on the reality of science studies.* Cambridge, MA: Harvard University Press.

McCarthy, L. P., & Gerring, J. P. (1994). Revising psychiatry's charter document: DSM-IV. *Written Communication, 11*(2), 147–191.

Middleton, M., Hess, A., Endres, D., & Senda-Cook, S. (2015). *Participatory critical rhetoric: Theoretical and methodological foundations for studying rhetoric in situ.* Lanham, MD: Lexington Books. Retrieved from http://ebookcentral.proquest.com/lib/jmu/detail.action?docID=4306502, doi:10.1177/0741088394011002001.

Miller, E. (2019). Too fat to be president? Chris Christie and fat stigma as rhetorical disability. *Rhetoric of Health & Medicine, 2*(1), 60–87. doi:10.5744/rhm.2019.1003.

Mittal, D., M. D., Sullivan, G., M. D., Chekuri, L., M. D., Allee, E., M. A., & Corrigan, P. W. (2012). Empirical studies of self-stigma reduction strategies: A critical review of the literature. *Psychiatric Services, 63*(10), 974–981. doi:10.1176/appi.ps.201100459.

Mol, A. (1998). Ontological politics: A word and some questions. *Sociological Review, 46*(S1), 74–89. doi:10.1111/1467-954X.46.s.5.

Mol, A. (2000). Pathology and the clinic: An ethnographic presentation of two atheroscleroses. In M. Lock, A. Young, & A. Cambrosio (Eds.), *Living and working with the new medical technologies* (pp. 82–102). Cambridge, UK: Cambridge University Press. doi:10.1017/CBO9780511621765.005.

Mol, A. (2002). *The body multiple: Ontology in medical practice*. Durham, NC: Duke University Press.

Mol, A., & Law, J. (2004). Embodied action, enacted bodies: The example of hypoglycemia. *Body & Society, 10*(2–3), 43–62.

Negrini, A., Corbière, M., Fortin, G., & Lecomte, T. (2014). Psychosocial well-being construct in people with severe mental disorders enrolled in supported employment programs. *Community Mental Health Journal Online, 50*(8), 932–942. doi:10.1007/s10597-014-9717-8.

Ono, K. A., & Sloop, J. M. (1995). The critique of vernacular discourse. *Communication Monographs, 62*(1), 19–46. doi:10.1080/03637759509376346.

Pescosolido, B. (2013). The public stigma of mental illness: What do we think; what do we know; what can we prove? *Journal of Health and Social Behavior, 54*(1), 1–21. doi:10.1177/0022146512471197.

Pescosolido, B., Martin, J. K., Long, J. S., Medina, T. R., Phelan, J. C., & Link, B. G. (2010). 'A disease like any other'? A decade of change in public reactions to schizophrenia, depression, and alcohol dependence. *The American Journal of Psychiatry, 167*, 1321–1230. doi:10.1176/appi.ajp.2010.09121743.

Popham, S. L. (2014). Hybrid disciplinarity: Métis and *ethos* in juvenile mental health electronic records. *Journal of Technical Writing and Communication, 44*(3), 329–344. doi:10.2190/TW.44.3.f.

Prendergast, C. (2001). On the rhetoric of mental disability. In J. Wilson (Ed.), *Embodied rhetoric: Disability in language and culture* (pp. 47–60). Carbondale, SC: Southern Illinois University Press.

Price, M. (2011). *Mad at school: Rhetorics of mental disability and academic life*. Lansing, MI: University of Michigan Press.

Pryal, K. R. G. (2010). The genre of the mood memoir and the *ethos* of psychiatric disability. *Rhetoric Society Quarterly, 40*(5), 479–501. doi:10.1080/02773945.2010.516304.

Reynolds, J. F. (2008). The rhetoric of mental health care. In B. Heifferon & S. C. Brown (Eds.), *Rhetoric of healthcare: Essays toward a new disciplinary inquiry* (pp. 149–157). Creskill, NJ: Hampton Press.

Reynolds, J. F. (2018). A short history of mental health rhetoric research (MHRR). *Rhetoric of Health & Medicine, 1*(1–2), 1–18. doi:10.5744/rhm.2018.1003.

Reynolds, J. F., & Mair, D. (1989). Patient records in the mental health disciplines. *Journal of Technical Writing and Communication, 19*(3), 245–254. doi:10.2190/2DE2-BUNG-VQEJ-FQ4G.

Reynolds, N. (1993). *Ethos* as location: New sites for understanding discursive authority. *Rhetoric Review, 11*(2), 325–338. doi:10.1080/07350199309389009.

Rusch, N., Müller, M., Lay, B., Corrigan, P. W., Zahn, R., Schönenberger, T., . . . Rössler, W. (2014). Emotional reactions to involuntary psychiatric hospitalization and stigma-related stress among people with mental illness. *Quality of Life Research, 264*(1), 35–43. doi:10.1007/s00406-013-0412-5.

Sangren, P. S. (1988). "Rhetoric and the authority of ethnography: Postmodernism and the social reproduction of texts." *Current Anthropology, 29*(3), 405–435. doi:10.1086/203652.

Segal, J. Z. (2003). Introduction scientific *ethos*: Authority, authorship, and trust in sciences. *Configurations, 11*(2), 137–144. doi:10.1353/con.2004.0023.

Segal, J. Z. (2005). *Health and the rhetoric of medicine*. Carbondale, SC: Southern Illinois University Press.

Thompson, R. (2004). Trauma and the rhetoric of recovery: A discourse analysis of the virtual healing journal of child sexual abuse survivors. *JAC, 24*(3), 653–675.

Thorvilson, M. J., & Copeland, A. J. (2018). Incompatible with care: Examining trisomy 18 medical discourse and families' counter-discourse for recuperative *ethos*. The Jour*nal of Medical Humanities, 39*(3), 349–360. doi:10.1007/s10912-017-9436-6.

Yergeau, M. (2017). *Authoring autism: On rhetoric and neurological queerness*. Durham, NC: Duke University Press. doi:10.1215/9780822372189.

6 Conclusion

Toward a Methodology for Studying Everyday *Ethos* in Clinical Settings

A Meditation on the Impact Diagnosis Has on Day-to-Day Life—An Occasion for Vindication or Stigma?

Karen,[1] a participant in the interview study described in Chapter 3, arrived in an ER at four in the morning with debilitating pain due to advanced endometriosis. A single mother, she had her two young children in tow. She was sure that she'd be taken seriously. Wouldn't the doctor realize that the pain would need to be quite severe for her to bring her small children with her to the emergency department in the middle of the night? When her pain was brushed off with a "Did you try an Advil?," she was sure that her gender impacted the care she received. Her assessment is well supported in the literature, which is clear that "women's pain reports are taken less seriously, their pain is discounted as being psychic or nonexistent, and their medication is less adequate than treatment given to men" (Samulowitz, Gremyr, Eriksson, & Hensing, 2018).

Karen's story illustrates a major premise of this book: that erroneous beliefs about a person's credibility—too often built out of the insidious energies of stigma and bias—can have dire consequences in health and medical contexts and beyond. As Chapter 2 demonstrated, for example, when a person is assumed to lack credibility because of demographic factors, particularly when power dynamics are added into the equation, the potential for inappropriate care is great. Another underlying theme of this book that deserves some concluding reflection is that diagnosis can be a very good thing or a very bad thing, but rarely is it values-neutral. When a person's physical symptoms have been summarily misattributed to psychological causes, missed opportunities for appropriate care follow, and avoidable progressions of disease or even preventable death are possible. In such cases, obtaining an accurate diagnosis such that the actual etiologies are explored and targeted becomes enormously important. As Chapter 3 made clear, diagnosis also brings relief in the form of an explanation for suffering—particularly for those who've been told that their symptoms are "all in their head."

Diagnosis, of course, gives a name to a set of symptoms, legitimizes them, and offers patients ways to seek out and leverage information and support from those with the same or similar condition. When a care provider renders a diagnosis, they are essentially saying, "What you are experiencing is *real*. It has a *name*." Once there *is* a name for a set of symptoms, too, the door opens for the patient to network with others with the same condition—an opportunity that has been greatly enhanced via new media (McKinley, 2019; Pengilly, 2019). Relatedly, having a name for a condition also helps a person to hone the health literacy skills necessary to gather as much information as possible on potential treatments and interventions. Diagnoses come with international classification of diseases (ICD) codes for which insurance policies can be billed for specific tests and treatments under Current Procedural Terminology (CPT) codes.[2] They also come with lifestyle change suggestions and, quite often, patient education materials. These textual practices, of course, are legitimizing. Regardless of prognosis, then, diagnosis can bring agency and options, as it offers opportunities to make strategic decisions.

For these reasons, diagnosis can even be read as empowering and life-altering—particularly for those who've been what I call "diagnostically unmoored" in Chapter 3 (or left without an accurate explanation for suffering). Indeed, being undiagnosed or misdiagnosed can lead to real feelings of despair, loneliness, and hopelessness. It is for these reasons that women like Lisa Smirl (those who've been misdiagnosed with symptoms "in their heads") are often enormously grateful for a physical diagnosis—even when that diagnosis is a terminal disease from which they might have been saved had they been accurately diagnosed sooner (Duff, 2012). The symbolic importance and material impact of diagnosis cannot, thus, be overstated. Undoubtedly, too, a diagnosis of a physical disease helps credibility when a person is finally found to not, after all, have symptoms that are merely "in their head."

That said, not all physical diagnoses are vindicating. Some diagnoses are actually quite stigmatizing, particularly when lifestyle factors are blamed for the onset of disease, as in lung cancer or type 2 diabetes—both of which are regularly blamed on lifestyle factors or character flaws (Cataldo, Jahan, & Pongquan, 2010; Chapple, Ziebland, & McPherson, 2004; Gonzalez & Jacobsen, 2012; Tak-Ying Shiu, Kwan, & Wong, 2003; Teixeira & Budd, 2010; Winkley et al., 2015). The same can be said for diagnoses of contested conditions, such as fibromyalgia and chronic fatigue syndrome, both of which are characterized as being "difficult to diagnose and having an elusive etiology and no clear-cut treatment strategy" and, thus, are likely to carry significant stigma (Åsbring, & Närvänen, 2002, p. 148). Indeed, as the film *Unrest* made clear, such conditions are quite frequently believed to be psychogenic in nature since so little is known about them, and the journey to diagnosis, as well as the quest to find effective treatment, is arduous (Dryden & Brea, 2017). Explained McInnis, Matheson, and Anisman (2014):

> Because the causes of these illnesses are unknown and objective diagnostic methods are vague, they are often viewed suspiciously. Indeed, affected individuals are often thought to be malingering, which might further impair wellbeing.
>
> (p. 602)

Thus, beyond the assumption that the symptoms are "all in your head," diagnoses of contested conditions can lead to other problems with credibility, such as the notion that the patient is simply lazy or looking for attention. Indeed, having a diagnosis of a condition that is complex, underdefined, and understudied can lead to some major issues with credibility. Phantom limb pain (PLP), another condition that is shrouded in etiological mystery, can also bring on problems with self-image and stigma, as claiming to have feeling in the missing limb is to be doubly undone in a rhetorical *ethotic* sense. When a person has an obvious physical difference, such as an amputated limb, their inability to thrive in everyday life might be misattributed to personal shortcomings rather than be attributed, as it should, to deficiencies in built environments and accommodations. As Chapter 4 emphasizes, too, such persons undoubtedly know much more about their own bodies and experiences than they are given credit for, yet those who study their ailments are routinely given the final word on their realities.

Perhaps no physical conditions, though, carry quite the same level of stigma as do mental illnesses. Indeed, those with serious, chronic mental health-related diagnoses, such as the men and women with schizophrenia and bipolar diagnoses I was fortunate enough to spend time with to conceptualize "recuperative *ethos*" and "agile epistemologies" in Chapter 5, suffer myriad personal, social, and material consequences that come with mental illness stigma and the attendant near-total loss of credibility (Corrigan & Kleinlein, 2005; Link, Yang, Phelan, & Collins, 2004; Rüsch, Angermeyer, & Corrigan, 2005). Just as a diagnosis of a physical disease can, in some cases, mean an upshot to credibility for those whose symptoms have been doubted, a diagnosis of a mental health problem almost always means a major challenge to credibility. These two things, of course, are heavily related—the idea that a person's physical symptoms have no causes is essentially a diagnosis of a mental health problem and, thus, also carries stigma.

As Chapter 5 argued, too often, those with diagnoses such as schizophrenia and bipolar lose stable employment, intimate partnerships, and engaged communities, following what are often highly stigmatizing mental health "episodes"[3] and diagnoses—particularly if these experiences include psychiatric hospitalization. There is a strong link between these poignant personal, professional, and social losses and the loss of credibility that accompanies these mental health diagnoses.

Wrapped up in these realities are the too-often-underexamined sociological dimensions of diagnosis (Jutel, 2009), which call attention to the realities of diagnosis as quite comparable to reflections in distortion mirrors rather than to objective takes on what is happening with a person's body and mind (Reynolds, 2019). One major consideration in the landscape of the sociology of diagnosis is the difference between illness and disease as is discussed briefly in Chapter 5. This distinction, described in Kleinman (1988), made it clear that illnesses are problems a person faces in everyday life in the form of symptoms. "Illness" is, thus, a highly individual experience, while disease "is framed by the biological, rather than the personal" (Jutel, 2009, p. 287). Having a diagnosable disease, since it is considered a biological construct, might legitimize the experience of illness. Problematically, though, the experiences of suffering that would constitute an "illness" are not always legitimized once they are deemed due to "diseases," as is clear above in the discussion of fibromyalgia and chronic fatigue syndrome. In the case of mental health conditions, moreover, a diagnosis can pathologize certain behaviors as diseased while also delineating "normal" behavior (Reynolds, 2008, 2018; Reynolds, Mair, & Fischer, 1995; Reynolds & Mairs, 1989). In the same way, those with symptoms believed to be "in their heads" or those complaining of symptoms for which no cause can be found can be erroneously believed to be delusional or attention-seeking.

When those with mental health diagnoses, contested diagnoses, disabilities, or unexplained symptoms are regarded as highly unreliable, the damage to their *ethos* can lead to worthwhile persons being cut off from public life. In such cases, not only do individual lives become embroiled in unlivable conditions, but the entire human community is deprived of these individuals' full potential contributions. In the research participants I was able to interact with in real time, as well as in those who were reanimated on blue cardstock remarkably well preserved from the 19th century, there are countless narratives of pain, suffering, isolation, inertia, and abandonment. In my estimation, most of this misery is traceable to stigma and bias, and the layers of complexity that account for these prejudices can seem dauntingly impenetrable. What role, I've asked, does credibility play in all of this? How can theories of *ethos* help to clarify these participants' everyday attempts to fight back? To address these questions, I've also had to ask what a methodology for studying everyday *ethos* in health and medical contexts might look like.

Such a task is a difficult one, as the state of feeling unwell in body or mind (or both) is amorphous, shifting, and ephemeral. Yet diagnosis of disease imbues these complex ontologies with a false sense of certainty and finality. While diagnosis "guides medical care" and organizes "the clinical picture" in ways that "determine intervention," it is also "interpretive," as it "provides structure to a narrative of dysfunction . . . and imposes official order, sorting out the real from the imagined, the valid from the feigned, the significant from the insignificant" (Jutel, 2009, p. 279). In a sleight of hand, it makes a complex, dynamic portrait of human experience static and settled. This book intervenes in these processes by examining the vernacular utterances of participants discussing their health histories in the context of everyday life. It also does so by examining, in the case of Chapter 5, the everyday talk of those transitioning from inpatient mental healthcare settings to community settings. In so doing, it elevates these shifting discursive behaviors to the level of data worthy of serious study and theories-building.

Toward a Methodology for Studying Everyday *Ethos* in Clinical Settings

This book has used theories of rhetorical *ethos* and ephemeral rhetorics of the everyday/rhetorics of the vernacular to examine patients' strategies for building and rebuilding credibility in clinical and related contexts. Thus, it has worked toward a methodology, and the next section of this chapter articulates that approach and hopes, in this way, to contribute to burgeoning scholarship on efficacious and ethical research practices in rhetoric of health and medicine (RHM). For example, De Hertogh (2018) highlighted "ethical concerns regarding consent, privacy, and circulation" to "remind us that not all health data should be shared or published" (p. 499), and Bivens (2017) asked readers to consider "microwithdrawals of consent" such that participants' agency would be accounted for in ways that exceed typical institutional review board (IRB) protocols on informed consent processes. Still, Scott and Melonçon (2017) lamented that "too little attention is given to documenting and explaining decisions made during the research process" (p. 10). The methodology for studying everyday *ethos* in clinical settings that I outline below has four constituent elements I will enumerate with explanations and applications for everyday research process decision-making:

- everyday inspiration, exigence, and affect
- open, emergent, hybrid methods
- creativity and hopefulness in analysis, and
- humility and confidence in researcher subjectivities.

Below, I elaborate on each of these elements such that other researchers interested in adapting similar approaches for their own work might use it as something of a very flexible roadmap.

Everyday Inspiration, Exigence, and Affect

Like many in RHM and beyond, I've used everyday life as a source of inspiration for the research projects that make up this book. Indeed, many in RHM and similar fields of study are "swept up into [research] topics that dominate . . . day-to-day life," so that "considering these personal-relational issues through rhetorical lenses feels somewhat inescapable" (Molloy et al., 2018, p. 353). This inevitability offers unique affordances to do with the differences between researching about personal health and medical realities versus writing about them in confessional narrative form. *Writing about* health and medical experiences might lead to psycho-analytically framed narrative arcs that are suggestive of catharsis. Such compositions might feel restorative to write and might help others going through similar situations. However, despite the potential power of sharing your story in the hopes that it could help others, the focus on healing the self is arguably the strongest application (Pennebaker, 1997). What's more, writing your health and medical story—particularly if your role is/was caregiver—brings up a number of questions on the ethics of representation and disclosure worth serious meditation.[4] *Researching* personal health and medical contexts, though, can be a productive way to symbolically recast painful or even traumatic experiences in health and medical contexts into generative inquiries that might extend further beyond the self. Symbolically recasting highly personal health and medical experiences into research projects imbues them with passion and affect that are assets at the outset. Having personal stake in what you study also offers opportunity for private healing. Cultivating an openness to everyday life as inspiration for serious research in health and medicine and beyond allows researchers to articulate complex, multilayer questions—many of which are stumbled upon by accident or ushered into the scene uninvited. Some are highly personal and others are eruptions in affect and empathy that come with witnessing some near or remote suffering.

For example, in 2014, I happened to run into two colleagues from across campus at a Center for Faculty Innovation (CFI) event at my university. Coincidentally, both had been experiencing a range of troubling symptoms that year, such as fatigue, insomnia, digestive issues, and rapid heart rate. While the man was given a number of diagnostic tests to determine the causes, the woman was immediately prescribed Prozac—before any other causes were explored. That same year, I had developed my own debilitating stomach symptoms following a bout of gastroenteritis. After the initial 48 hours passed and the symptoms kept going, the texture of my day-to-day life changed drastically. I dropped 25 pounds in a matter of weeks. I dragged myself to work and slept under my desk between classes. I collapsed and went to sleep the minute I got home. I felt myself losing more and more weight. Staying hydrated took concerted effort.

Since we live in a thinness-obsessed culture, no one thought I looked sick. Friends congratulated me for getting back to "model weight."

Prior to that year, I'd never experienced symptoms for which no one could find an immediate cause. Over the course of months, the search for what was wrong became an all-consuming project involving a lot of symptoms checkers and web searches. I could not imagine how I would be able to keep my job or live my life or parent my child without figuring out what was making me so sick. Readers who've had mysterious symptoms and readers with chronic illnesses know such experiences all too well. In the emergency room, in an urgent care setting, in a gastroenterologist's office, I asked various providers what I thought was a pretty obvious question in my case: Could my experiences be related to my mental health? Since I was 34 at the time, they asked about my medical history. When I reported no previous mental health issues, they all said I was too old to develop issues severe enough to cause these symptoms now—even when I shared that I have a close family member with a chronic mental illness—the person whose experiences inspired my earlier research at the clubhouse described in Chapter 5. "Aren't these things, like, hereditary?" I'd asked.

An upper endoscopy, a colonoscopy, a stool study, a lot of blood work, and many months later, I was diagnosed with post-infectious irritable bowel syndrome (IBS)—a condition that can persist for years, but often eventually goes away. The doctor I saw described this as an entirely physical condition. However, explaining how physical and mental health collide to cause post-infectious IBS, Thabane and Marshall (2009) explained that "an exposure to pathogenic organisms disrupts intestinal barrier function, alters neuromuscular function and triggers chronic inflammation which sustain IBS symptoms" (p. 3591). While "the severity of the acute enteric infection" is one risk factor for developing post-infectious IBS, another is "psychological disorders" (Thabane & Marshall, 2009, p. 3592). When the gastroenterologist rendered this diagnosis, he said the only treatment was Imodium and other over-the-counter stomach medications, that he was sorry the symptoms were such a "nuisance," and that I could expect the condition to last months to years. "Huh," I responded, "How is that even a thing?!" While not great news, I was relieved to know what was happening.

I also left convinced that I *did* need mental health help if I was in for months to years of these symptoms, so I got a very good therapist. That therapist helped me to cope with the anxiety and panic attacks that came with the fear of going to public places due to terror that I'd, once again, end up making multiple trips to the bathroom before sweating and ultimately fainting. These experiences left me feeling very concerned for those with severe symptoms for which no one could find a cause and for those, like my colleague, whose physical symptoms were rapidly dismissed as "in her head."

My experiences and the experiences of my colleagues left me with a lot of questions that seemed related to my ongoing interest in mental health and rhetoric. Why were my female colleague's providers so convinced that there was nothing physically wrong with her and that she had anxiety? Why were my care providers so convinced that nothing mental health-related was going on with me? From her descriptions of what she was experiencing, I certainly thought she needed to figure out the physical cause. In contrast and paradoxically, I felt for my male colleague, as he did have anxiety, and that anxiety was greatly exacerbated by unnecessary medical tests. These experiences also converged with my ongoing interest in the role rhetorical *ethos* plays in patient empowerment. I found myself increasingly drawn to ailments of bodies and minds and the permeable boundaries between them, which led me to examine phantom limb pain. I found myself fixated on the idea that my own credibility in clinical conversations might even have been strangely bolstered by my admission that I believed I was having mental health-related symptoms.[5] These experiences, of course, led me to study patients' everyday strategies for establishing and repairing credibility in health and medical settings.

This brief account, I hope, makes it clear that part of a methodology for studying everyday *ethos* in health and medicine is allowing for the possibility that your everyday life might gift you with opportunities for angles and layers to examine, but being open to such shifts in your research trajectory means letting go of the idea of a fixed and permanent research agenda. Allowing everyday life to infiltrate your research agenda also means finding ways to manage the affect that accompanies the choices to focus scholarly attention on issues and topics that already consume your personal and even spiritual attention. Managing affect, diffuse in all areas of this kind of research, is, thus, another needed consideration for those doing this work—particularly when you and/or your loved ones are part of a highly stigmatized health community. Bearing witness to more suffering along those same lines through interacting with participants and data can mean tripping into a well of grief related to some highly personal memories or associations in the context of the professional activity of data collection. Still, intensity begets more intensity. These emotional land mines might, ironically, be researcher assets. They lead to heightened attunement to the research scene and to participants.

Open, Emergent, Hybrid Methods

As the previous section demonstrated, generative, rich, affectively potent research questions can emerge from everyday life in the form of what a person directly experiences and what they witness. Since day-to-day life can be fraught with uncertainty, it often yields research directions that are quite difficult to predict very far in advance. Likewise, once questions are established, of course, they are not really fixed, but are, instead, suggestive of myriad possible directions. Such shifting questions are often best answered with everyday, ephemeral data, and such data very often demand hybrid methods to gather. Developing open, emergent, hybrid methods often means borrowing and adapting social science and humanities methods of inquiry, and such approaches were used in the projects examined in this book. The strongest example of a hybrid approach among the projects featured in this book is in Chapter 5. That project began as a broad inquiry into the everyday rhetorical strategies of a population—chronic mental illness patients—who'd been too often characterized as totally devoid of rhetoricity. That said, many obvious issues with access and ethics were at play. Thus, I used many aspects of rhetorical ethnography, but I needed to add in aspects of naturalistic inquiry found in anthropology such that I was not claiming to really "participant-observe," but to simply "observe."

In the same way, I chose to create a survey instrument through which participant recruitment might be accomplished with a difficult-to-define population. I also chose to use interviews for the study featured in Chapter 3 because I wanted to establish a density of patients' experiences arguing effectively for their credibility after their symptoms were doubted. Interviewing allowed me to play a bit of a temporal trick as it gave me insight into decades-worth of 68 people's experiences with clinical conversations over the course of only a year and a half of interviewing. Gaining that amount of data related directly to my research question would quite literally have taken decades had I not done these interviews. Still, I call the approach hybrid because the interviews basically asked speakers to recreate these clinical conversations and to offer their own analysis of their credibility. I asked the speakers to bring me to the exam rooms they'd been in over the courses of their lives without having to invade those spaces and without having to find ways to identify a site where misdiagnosis of psychogenic symptoms related to stigma and bias is a common occurrence—a task that felt impossible. In both cases, the questions were open in terms of what might be learned, yet specific in terms of who I wanted to learn from. Similarly, I used some archival methods with the PLP surveys, yet I ultimately chose to treat the data like contemporary health surveys—a move that helped me to identify prescience in the men's words. In all of three cases, the hybridity in methods led to extraordinary data, and flexibility led to these hybrid approaches.

Creativity and Hopefulness in Analysis

Once hybrid methods have given way to rich data, it is advantageous to gather up that ephemera and examine it for traces, for residues, and, ultimately, for new theories. Seeking theories of everyday *ethos* from ephemeral data means engaging with various existing theories of *ethos* and of other generative rhetorical terms, such *doxa* and *metis*. It also means, though, allowing the data to suggest a new theory or set of theories out of the energetic patterns you see in the data you have. Since this work is unpredictable, too, there is a need to accept the data you have even if it is quite different from what you imagined getting.

Dierckx de Casterlé, Gastmans, Bryon, and Denier (2012) emphasized the role of intuition and creativity in qualitative research, and allowing for the possibility that something extraordinary is happening in all of the things that are so easily missed in the local rhythms of day-to-day lives, in gestures, voices, tones, and textures or utterances that come and go, can lend itself especially well to creative analysis. An imaginative and open approach to data analysis is necessary for this kind of data, as it cannot simply be treated as some variation on sanctioned texts. Indeed, "vernacular discourse cannot be examined as bits and pieces of hegemonic culture itself but, instead, should be analyzed as a whole new hybrid, through its own conditions of emergence" (Ono & Sloop, 1995, p. 40).

Performing this kind of analysis means suspending disbelief a bit, as I did when I approached analyses in Chapter 4. That chapter, of course, describes a project for which there was not very much extant data, yet the data that were there were incredibly compelling. Likewise, in Chapter 5, after coding for "recuperative *ethos*," the data I ended up coding as "agile epistemologies" evolved from the leftover, yet still quite intriguing data. Lingering with data that speaks to you, yet is not quite voluminous or that does not fit the initial analysis framework, is appropriate for this kind of research.

Notably, Chapter 2 shares literature on anchoring bias on the part of care providers and notes that this phenomenon occurs when a doctor is unwilling to accept a diagnosis that differs from their initial judgment. In the same way, a methodology for studying everyday *ethos* in health and medical settings requires a tentativeness and an ability to scrap wide swaths of analysis if some new data enters into the analytic scene, or if some new way of seeing that data becomes available via the researcher's own everyday experiences. Importantly, layers of affect can accumulate when a researcher is faced with everyday health and medical realties that are deeply unjust. Rather than eschewing that affect in favor of some feigned objective way of doing analysis, embracing it as an embodied part of the important work of elevating the significance of vernacular data can enrich the creativity in data analysis.

A final consideration for analyzing complex, ephemeral health and medical data is hopefulness. Research, asserted Tuhiwai Smith (2006), "began as a social, intellectual, and imaginative activity," so while it "has become disciplined and institutionalized with certain approaches empowered over others and accorded a legitimacy," it is important to remember that "it begins with human curiosity and a desire to solve problems. It is, at its core, an activity of hope" (p. 355). This disposition, drawn from decolonial research methodologies, is tremendously important in analyzing vernacular health and medical data from the perspective of rhetorical *ethos*. Attempting to elevate undervalued data means adapting an analytic mindset that is also on the margins.

Vernacular health and medical projects focused on rhetorical *ethos* are at their best when there is an implicit hope at the backdrop of analyses—a hope that the data matters and that the theories that emerge from it can also matter. Just as the data such projects generate might easily have slipped through the cracks of spatial and temporal realities, so too can these analyses feel tenuous and slippery. The researcher's vantage, though, is most astute when they are able to retain a sense of hope for what the work might do.

Humility and Confidence in Researcher Subjectivities

Finally, performing research on the everyday focused on *ethos* in clinical settings requires humility and confidence in equal measures. For one, as this book makes clear, there is a need to have confidence in one's ability to access unusual research sites—ones where those in hybrid fields between the humanities and social sciences might not ordinarily be present. A researcher must have confidence in the legitimacy of their field of study and the strength of the new knowledge it generates such that those working in the trenches with vulnerable patients, for example, and the patients themselves, will see that value and wish to contribute to the project. Likewise, performing creative data analysis requires confidence. It takes conviction to see evidence of a trace rhetorical tactic and to assert its truth or at least its possibility. Researchers must be confident that the data will speak to them.

Equally important is researcher humility. A humble researcher "respects differences, affirms similarities, and promotes an unknown place of emptiness between" for the research and the participants (SooHoo, 2013, p. 207). Chapter 4 argues that patients' contributions to research are too often undervalued and that analyses do not bear out the full potential of those contributions. Taking stock of this reality aids in the cultivation of humility in the researcher. Allowing for the possibility of exploratory findings requires humility. A tentativeness to the findings is a realistic stance as the vernacular discursive practices I gained access to are necessarily tainted by my presence. Indeed, humility, explained SooHoo (2013) "not only plays a role in the preparation of one's self for research with others, but it is also the sustaining force and space between the researcher and participants" (p. 208).

A thorough accounting of research subjectivities, highly necessary in this work, relates to the literature on implicit bias that appears in Chapter 2. Readers will recall that implicit bias occurs when a care provider becomes so attached to an initial diagnosis that they ignore other possibilities—even in the face of new evidence. This concept aptly captures the spirit of subconscious bias on the part of researchers. These biases can take the form of unwittingly undervaluing the data coming from vernacular sources, which could lead to missed opportunities for adding important new knowledges to a complex health and medical phenomenon. In the same way, researchers must be mindful of how they are representing participants and must hold back data that is too private to be shared. Thus, there are many stories left out of Chapters 3 and 5 in particular, as participants naturally shared more over the course of our everyday conversations than they'd want to see in print.

Another feature of a productive methodology for studying rhetorical *ethos* in health and medical contexts is the ability to articulate limitations. Thus, readers will note that each chapter takes on limitations directly. Taking stock of limitations often, then, leads to thoughts on what work might come next. In this book, my own assessment is that more work should be done in the area of credibility in everyday health and medicine in terms of physician *ethos* and its relation to concordance. Just as "there will be substantial social, economic and scientific costs if we cannot improve the diversity of our biomedical research workforce" (Economou, 2014, p. 1063), the consequences of lack of diversity in highly trained medical staff poses problems for patients. A second assertion is that more work is needed in the area of chemical dependency discourses within everyday rhetorical *ethos* frameworks. That said, potential new directions are multiple by design. While humility allows me to recognize that the flaws in this work are likely many, confidence lets me also see the work as valuable and generative—as paving the way for more and better work to come.

Summing Up

The framework offered in this chapter has been intentionally open-ended as there is a danger in overprescribing a methodological approach to unstable and shifting data. Indeed, "articulating a framework for studying and utilizing the vernacular must be malleable and able to change as conventions of the everyday are also continually changing" (Hauser & McClellen, 2009, p. 43).

In sum, this book has used a wide variety of ephemeral data to perform original theorizing toward several important goals:

- to ennoble what might otherwise be considered throwaway or trace material by elevating it to the level of data worthy of serious study (and, thus, add to literature on rhetorics of the vernacular and rhetorics of the everyday)
- to provide a model for similar studies of ephemeral health and medical data drawn from patients' everyday rhetorical contributions (and, thus, add to mental health rhetoric research [MHRR] work that is already taking such things quite seriously), and

- to build a flexible set of methodologies and theories that might lead to future study in diverse health and medical contexts (and, thus, help other researchers to elevate, legitimize, and theorize complex data).

In modest form, it has attempted to make a generative contribution to efforts in the humanities to offer hybrid models of scholarship that speak across and between disciplinary lines. It is my sincerest hope that other studies will take energy and inspiration from the studies in this book and that those studies will exceed the work herein.

Notes

1. Readers will recognize Karen's story from the discussion of emphasizing day-to-day impairment to elicit physician empathy in Chapter 3.
2. In the US, Medicare can be billed under the Healthcare Common Procedure Coding System (HCPCS) codes.
3. Indeed, even the notion of a mental health "episode" implies a time away from "real" or "regular" life.
4. Of course ethics of representation are still highly important in research in terms of how researchers represent participants.
5. My experience made me think I'd find this same pattern in the data I collected for Chapter 3, but there was only one participant out of the 68 who'd similarly found that care providers believed they did not have mental health problems because they said out loud that they feared they might.

References

Åsbring, P., & Närvänen, A. (2002). Women's experiences of stigma in relation to chronic fatigue syndrome and fibromyalgia. *Qualitative Health Research, 12*(2), 148–160. doi:10.1177/104973230201200202.

Bivens, K. M. (2017). Rhetorically listening for micro withdrawals of consent in research practice. In J. B. Scott & L. Melonçon (Eds.), *Methodologies for the rhetoric of health and medicine* (pp. 138–156). New York: Routledge.

Cataldo, J. K., Jahan, T. M., & Pongquan, V. L. (2010). The European journal of oncology nursing. *European Journal of Oncology Nursing, 14*(2), iv. doi:10.1016/S1462-3889(10)00044-X.

Chapple, A., Ziebland, S., & McPherson, A. (2004). Stigma, shame, and blame experienced by patients with lung cancer: Qualitative study. *BMJ (Clinical Research Ed.), 328*(7454), 1470. doi:10.1136/bmj.38111.639734.7C.

Corrigan, P. W., & Kleinlein, P. (2005). The impact of mental illness stigma. In P. W. Corrigan (Ed.), *On the stigma of mental illness: Practical strategies for research and social change* (pp. 11–44). Washington, DC: American Psychological Association. http://dx.doi.org/10.1037/10887-001

De Hertogh, L. B. (2018). Feminist digital research methodology for rhetoricians of health and medicine. *Journal of Business and Technical Communication, 32*(4), 480–503. https://doi.org/10.1177/1050651918780188.

Dierckx de Casterlé, B., Gastmans, C., Bryon, E., & Denier, Y. (2012). QUAGOL: A guide for qualitative data analysis. *International Journal of Nursing Studies, 49*(3),

360–371. Retrieved from www.sciencedirect.com/science/article/pii/S0020748
911003671

Dryden, L. (Producer), & Brea, J. (Director). (2017). *Unrest.* [Video/DVD] Shella
Films. Retrieved from www.imdb.com/title/tt3268850/

Duff, L. (2012). And now some words from my friends: Lisa. Retrieved from https://out
livinglungcancer.com/2012/11/18/and-now-some-words-from-my-friends-lisa/

Economou, J. S. (2014). Gender bias in biomedical research. *Surgery, 156*(5),
1061–1065. doi:10.1016/j.surg.2014.07.005.

Gonzalez, B. D., & Jacobsen, P. B. (2012). Depression in lung cancer patients:
The role of perceived stigma. *Psycho-Oncology, 21*(3), 239–246. doi:10.1002/
pon.1882.

Hauser, G. A., & McClellen, E. D. (2009). Vernacular rhetoric and social movements: Performances of resistance in the rhetoric of the everyday. In S. M. Stevens &
P. M. Malesh (Eds.), *Active voices: Composing a rhetoric for social movements*
(pp. 23–46). Albany, NY: State University of New York Press. Retrieved from
http://ebookcentral.proquest.com/lib/jmu/detail.action?docID=3408354

Jutel, A. (2009). Sociology of diagnosis: A preliminary review. *Sociology of Health &
Illness, 31*(2), 278–299. doi:10.1111/j.1467-9566.2008.01152.x.

Kleinman, A. (1988). *The illness narratives: Suffering, healing, and the human
condition.* New York: Basic Books, Inc.

Link, B. G., Yang, L. H., Phelan, J. C., & Collins, P. Y. (2004). Measuring mental
illness stigma. *Schizophrenia Bulletin, 30*(3), 511–541. doi:10.1093/oxford-
journals.schbul.a007098.

McInnis, O. A., Matheson, K., & Anisman, H. (2014). Living with the unexplained: Coping, distress, and depression among women with chronic fatigue
syndrome and/or fibromyalgia compared to an autoimmune disorder. *Anxiety,
Stress, & Coping, 27*(6), 601–618. doi:10.1080/10615806.2014.888060.

McKinley, M. (2019). Analyzing PCOS discourses: Strategies for unpacking chronic
illness and taking action. *Women's health advocacy: Rhetorical ingenuity for the
21st century* (pp. 34–44). New York: Routledge. Retrieved from www.crcpress.
com/Womens-Health-Advocacy-Rhetorical-Ingenuity-for-the-21st-Century/
White-Farnham-Finer-Molloy/p/book/9780367192259

Molloy, C., Beemer, C., Bennett, J., Green, A., Johnson, J., Kessler, M., . . . Siegel-
Finer, B. (2018). A dialogue on possibilities for embodied methodologies in the
rhetoric of health & medicine. *Rhetoric of Health & Medicine, 1*(3–4), 349–371.
doi:10.5744/rhm.2018.1017.

Ono, K. A., & Sloop, J. M. (1995). The critique of vernacular discourse. *Communication Monographs, 62*(1), 19–46. doi:10.1080/03637759509376346.

Pengilly, C. (2019). Rhetorics of empowerment for managing lupus pain: Patient-to-
patient knowledge sharing in online health forums. In *Women's health advocacy:
Rhetorical ingenuity for the 21st century* (pp. 45–58). New York: Routledge.
Retrieved from www.crcpress.com/Womens-Health-Advocacy-Rhetorical-
Ingenuity-for-the-21st-Century/White-Farnham-Finer-Molloy/p/book/978036
7192259

Pennebaker, J. W. (1997). Writing about emotional experiences as a therapeutic
process. *Psychological Science, 8*(3), 162–166. https://doi.org/10.1111/j.1467-
9280.1997.tb00403.x.

Reynolds, F. (personal communication, June 13, 2019). Email on diagnosis as distortion mirror. Reynolds, J. F. (2018). A short history of mental health rhetoric

research (MHRR). *Rhetoric of Health & Medicine, 1*(1–2), 1–18. doi:10.5744/rhm.2018.1003.

Reynolds, J. F. (2008). The rhetoric of mental health care. In B. Heifferon & S. C. Brown (Eds.), *Rhetoric of healthcare: Essays toward a new disciplinary inquiry* (pp. 149–157). Creskill, NJ: Hampton Press.

Reynolds, J. F., & Mair, D. (1989). Patient records in the mental health disciplines. *Journal of Technical Writing and Communication, 19*(3), 245–254. doi:10.2190/2DE2-BUNG-VQEJ-FQ4G.

Reynolds, J. F., Mair, D. C., & Fischer, P. C. (1995). *Writing and reading mental health records: Issues and analysis in professional writing and scientific rhetoric*. Mahwah, NJ: L. Erlbaum Associates.

Rüsch, N., Angermeyer, M. C., & Corrigan, P. W. (2005). Mental illness stigma: Concepts, consequences, and initiatives to reduce stigma. *European Psychiatry, 20*(8), 529–539. doi:10.1016/j.eurpsy.2005.04.004.

Samulowitz, A., Gremyr, I., Eriksson, E., & Hensing, G. (2018). "Brave men" and "emotional women": A theory-guided literature review on gender bias in health care and gendered norms towards patients with chronic pain. *Pain Research & Management, 2018*, 6358624. doi:10.1155/2018/6358624.

Scott, J. B., & Melonçon, L. (Eds.). (2017). *Methodologies for the rhetoric of health and medicine*. New York: Routledge.

Smith, L. T. (2006). Choosing the margins: The role of research in indigenous struggles for social justice. In N. K. Denzin & M. D. Giardina (Eds.), *Qualitative inquiry and the conservative challenge* (pp. 151–173). Walnut Creek, CA: Left Coast Press.

SooHoo, S. (2013). Humility within culturally responsive methodologies. In M. Berryman, S. SooHoo, & A. Nevin (Eds.), *Culturally responsive methodologies* (pp. 199–219). Bingley, West Yorkshire, England: Emerald Group Publishing.

Tak-Ying Shiu, A., Kwan, J. J. Y., & Wong, R. Y. (2003). Social stigma as a barrier to diabetes self-management: Implications for multi-level interventions. *Journal of Clinical Nursing, 12*(1), 149–150. doi:10.1046/j.1365-2702.2003.00735.x.

Teixeira, M. E., & Budd, G. M. (2010). Obesity stigma: A newly recognized barrier to comprehensive and effective type 2 diabetes management. *Journal of the American Academy of Nurse Practitioners, 22*(10), 527–533. doi:10.1111/j.1745-7599.2010.00551.x.

Thabane, M., & Marshall, J. (2009). Post-infectious irritable bowel syndrome. *World Journal of Gastroenterology, 15*(29), 3591–3596. Retrieved from https://www.ncbi.nlm.nih.gov/pmc/articles/PMC2721231/

Winkley, K., Evwierhoma, C., Amiel, S. A., Lempp, H. K., Ismail, K., & Forbes, A. (2015). Patient explanations for non-attendance at structured diabetes education sessions for newly diagnosed type 2 diabetes: A qualitative study. *Diabetic Medicine, 32*(1), 120–128. doi:10.1111/dme.12556.

Index

Note: Page numbers in *italic* indicate a figure on the corresponding page. Footnotes are indicated by n.

For Product Safety Concerns and Information please contact our EU
representative GPSR@taylorandfrancis.com
Taylor & Francis Verlag GmbH, Kaufingerstraße 24, 80331 München, Germany

9 781032 176888